Anatomy for Problem Solving in Sports Medicine
The Back

First published by Nottingham University Press

This reissued original edition published 2023 by 5m Books Ltd www.5mbooks.com

British Library Cataloguing in Publication Data
Anatomy for Problem Solving in Sports Medicine: The Back
Prof. P. Harris and Dr. C. Ranson

ISBN 9781789183108

Disclaimer

Every reasonable effort has been made to ensure that the material in this book is true, correct, complete and appropriate at the time of writing. Nevertheless the publishers and the author do not accept responsibility for any omission or error, or for any injury, damage, loss or financial consequences arising from the use of the book. Views expressed in the articles are those of the author and not of the Editor or Publisher.

Typeset by Nottingham University Press, Nottingham

EU GPSR Authorised Representative
LOGOS EUROPE, 9 rue Nicolas Poussin, 17000, LA ROCHELLE, France
E-mail: Contact@logoseurope.eu

Anatomy for Problem Solving in Sports Medicine:

The Back

Philip F Harris MD , MSc , MB ChB
Emeritus Professor of Anatomy, University of Manchester, Tutor in Anatomy, University of Nottingham Medical School UK, past Visiting Professor, Centre for Sports Medicine, Queen's Medical Centre, University of Nottingham

Craig Ranson BSc, PGD, PhD
Lecturer in Sports and Exercise Medicine Cardiff Metropolitan University UWIC. Wales Rugby Team Physiotherapist and Member of the International Cricket Council Medical Committee.

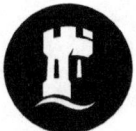

Nottingham
University Press

Acknowledgements

We wish to thank Sarah Keeling, Production Manager, Nottingham University Press for guiding us through the preparation of this book and for her unfailing forbearance in the face of frequent requests from the authors for additions and alterations. We are also grateful to Professor R.S.Harris and Dr Aditya Daftary for contributing radiological images and advice.

Special thanks are due to Dr Margaret Pratten, Associate Professor of Anatomy, for generously allowing access to facilities in the Department of Anatomy, School of Biomedical Sciences, University of Nottingham Medical School.

Foreword

Back injuries are amongst the most common causes of lost training and competition time for those participating in sport and the structural complexity of the region poses significant challenges to those involved in athletic back injury management. Accurate diagnosis and effective treatment requires a sound knowledge of the structural and functional anatomy of the back and its component parts.

Our purpose in writing this book is to present the anatomy in a manner that provides a foundation for solving 'real world' clinical problems. Examples of problems requiring such knowledge are presented throughout the text. Radiographic images of the type commonly encountered in sports medicine are included to facilitate the recognition and interpretation of injured or abnormal structures.

We are confident the book will be valuable to students and practitioners* involved in diagnosis, management and rehabilitation of back injuries in sport.

Prof. PF Harris
Dr. C Ranson
Nottingham, 2011

*Including Sports Medicine Physicians, Physiotherapists, Osteopaths, Chiropractors, Orthopaedic and Neuro-surgery trainees, Athletic Trainers and Rehabilitation Specialists.

Contents

INTRODUCTION

Because of its unique position in the body as a result of man's upright posture the back is particularly vulnerable to stresses and strains. All components of the back including bones, joints, ligaments, muscles and nerves are susceptible to damage. In the western world, back pain is one of the biggest causes of lost working days. This is reflected even more in the athletic environment with back injury being a major cause of lost training and playing time across a variety of sports. The back is exposed to traumatic injury in activities involving the risk of extremely high forces such as motorsports, parachute sports, tackling football codes (Rugby and Rugby League, Australian and American Football) and maximal weight lifting. Acute muscle strain, ligament disruption, and even fracture, joint dislocation and associated spinal cord or nerve injury may result. However, most incidences of back injury in sport are due to cumulative micro-trauma involving sustained or repeated stress applied to component tissues such as the trunk musculature, the inter-vertebral discs, the various joint complexes and the bony structure. For example, sports involving repeated or sustained trunk flexion, such as cycling and rowing (Perich *et al.*, 2011), have high incidences of intervertebral disc related pain whilst sports involving repeated back extension (often combined with rotation and side-flexion) such as gymnastics, golf, throwing and cricket fast bowling (Ranson *et al.*, 2010), butterfly and breaststroke swimming, have high rates of bony stress and zygapophyseal (facet) joint injury. As well as patho-anatomical causes, it is increasingly acknowledged that bio-psycho-social factors can play an important role in the incidence, severity and recurrence of back injury. Diagnosing and managing sport- related back injury therefore requires an intimate knowledge of the region's complex anatomical structures.

The back comprises the dorsal region of the neck together with the trunk from the shoulders down to the iliac crests and gluteal regions. The spinal column forms its core. Placed deeply within the column itself, and therefore vulnerable to spinal injuries, lies the spinal cord surrounded by the meninges and cerebrospinal fluid (CSF) in the subarachnoid space. Spinal nerves arising from the cord emerge through the intervertebral foramina to form the roots of nerve plexuses, the major ones of which supply the limbs. The spine is formed by a column of bony vertebrae, linked by joints and ligaments. Immediately adjacent and attached to the column are groups of intrinsic muscles responsible for spinal movements and stability and for controlling posture, particularly man's upright (standing) posture. More superficial (extrinsic) muscles connect the proximal parts of the upper limb and shoulder girdle, particularly the clavicle, scapula and humerus, with the spine.

POSTURE AND CURVATURES

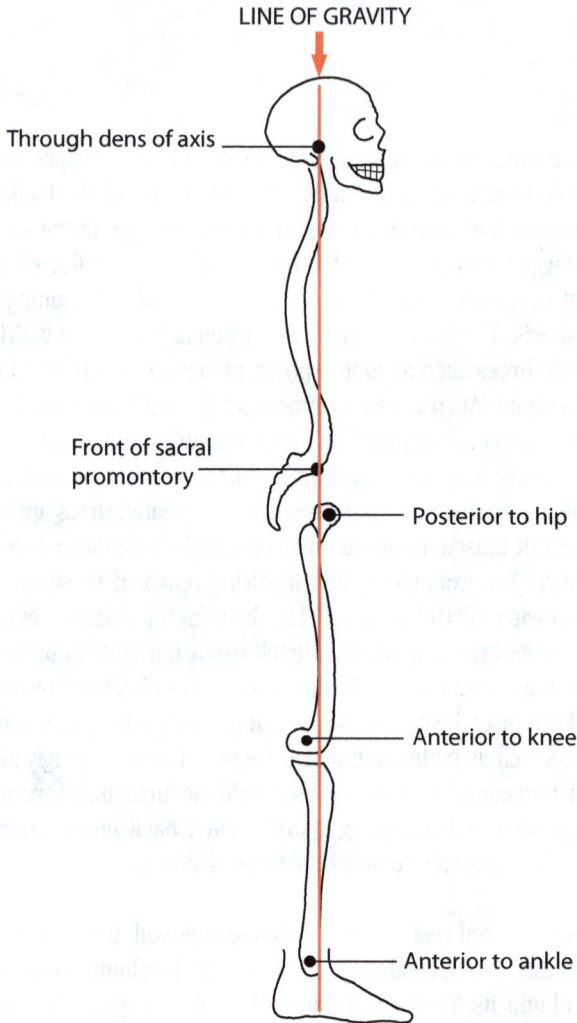

LINE OF GRAVITY

Through dens of axis

Front of sacral promontory

Posterior to hip

Anterior to knee

Anterior to ankle

Figure 1. The line of gravity in the upright posture

In the upright posture gravity acts behind the hip (Figure 1), causing the trunk to tilt backwards at the hip. This is resisted by tension in the strong iliofemoral ligament on the front of the hip joint. The knee joint also tends to overextend and this is resisted by tension in the collateral and anterior cruciate ligaments. At the ankle gravity tends to extend the joint and this is countered by contraction of the strong triceps surae muscle group (gastrocnemius and soleus) acting on the Achilles tendon to produce plantar flexion. It also tends to displace the tibia and fibula forwards on the dome of the talus. This is resisted by tension in the posterior components of the collateral ligaments.

Although the foetus can move in the amniotic sac and the head may occasionally extend, in general the foetal spine develops in a mostly flexed position. After birth as posture changes to an upright position i.e. sitting and standing, this leads to development of the secondary curvatures of the spine (Figure 2). Much of the curvature is due to the wedge-shape of the intervertebral discs and to a lesser extent of the vertebral bodies themselves. The S-shape of the curvatures has been interpreted to allow cushioning of vertical compression forces, for instance, those exerted during walking, running and jumping, or in falling from a height onto the feet.

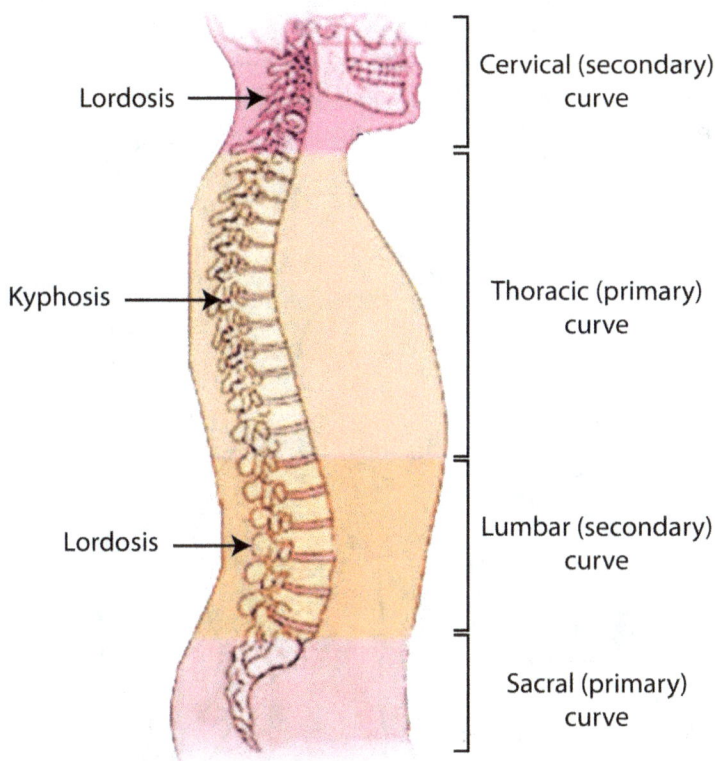

Figure 2. The normal curvatures of the spine

Excessive acceleration and deceleration forces, commonly encountered in motor-sports, may injure the cervical spine. Vertebral body fractures may be due to direct trauma or falls during, for example, contact or combat sports, or equestrian activities. Fractures and fracture-dislocations may result from forced flexion, which commonly damages the T5 or T6 vertebra. Vertical trauma along the spine resulting from falls onto the feet or head often converts to a flexion fracture at the level of T9 - L2 vertebra. The coccyx may be damaged by direct force. Falls during climbing and parachute based sports are often sources of these types of injuries.

A small amount of lumbar lordosis is normal in the female. Abnormal curvatures are shown in Figures 3 and 4. Lateral curvatures (scoliosis) in the thoraco-lumbar region especially when they occur in female adolescents may be masked by compensatory curvature more proximally in the thoraco-cervical region. This tendency requires careful monitoring especially in young female athletes involved in sports requiring repeated lumbar extension e.g. gymnastics and diving, due to risk of spondylolysis and progression to spondylolysthesis. Moreover, any sports involving repeated deviation of the spine to one side can result in unequal pressure on the growth end-plate of the vertebral body and this could trigger asymmetrical growth in the plate and consequently abnormal curvature. Excessive kyphosis may be combined with scoliosis. On the compression side where there is crowding of the ribs, thoracic space is reduced leading to lung compression, increased resistance to pulmonary blood flow and subsequent right heart pressure over-load. Paralympic athletes competing in wheelchair or seated events are particularly susceptible.

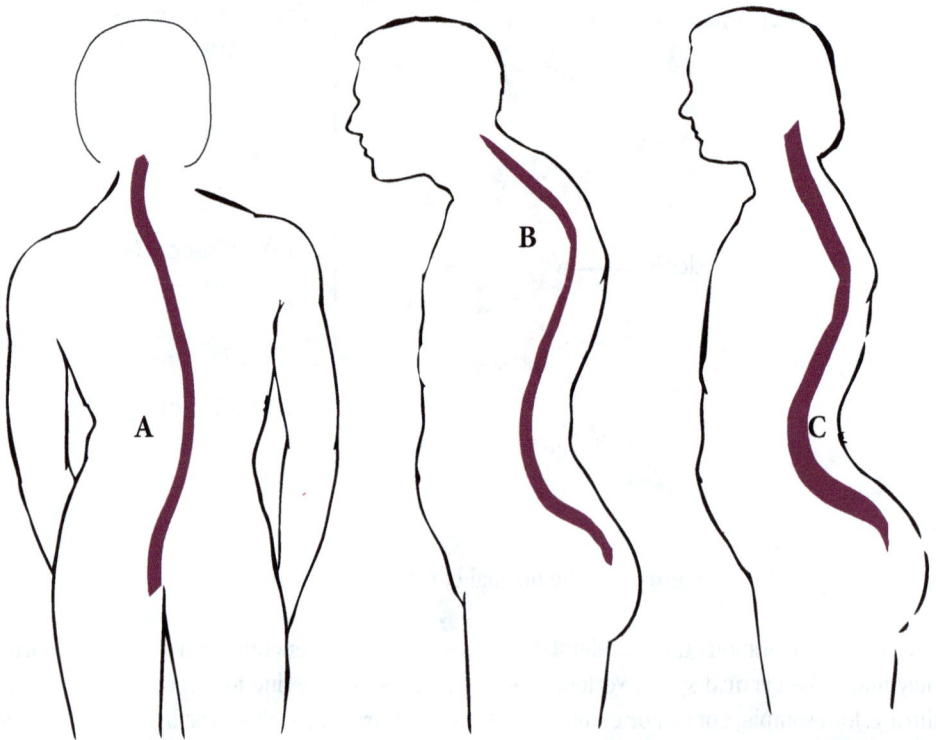

Figure 3. Abnormal spinal curvatures.
(A) Scoliosis (B) Hyper-kyphosis (C) Hyper-lordosis

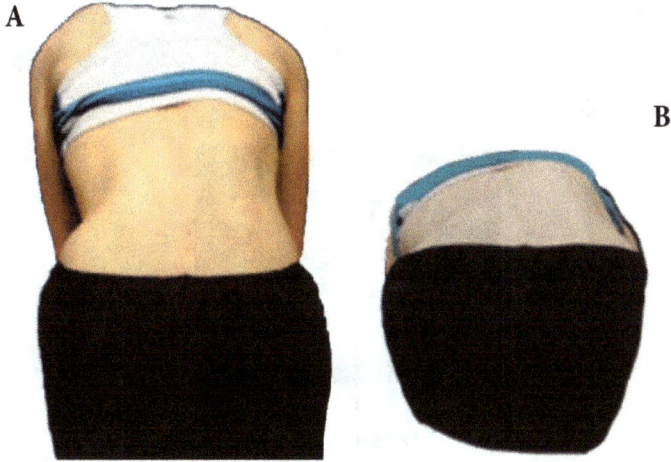

Figure 4A. Kypho-scoliosis in an athlete
Figure 4B. Asymmetry of thoracic wall contour revealed when the trunk is fully flexed

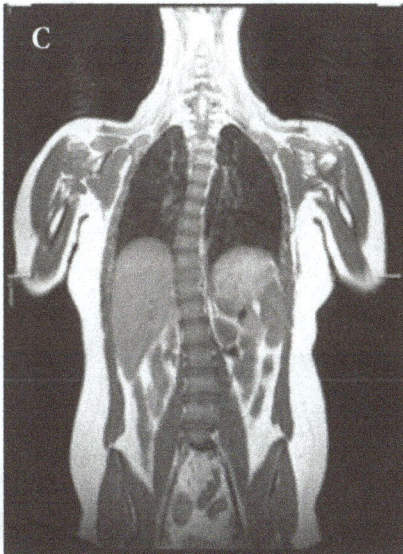

Figure 4C. Coronal MRI scan showing kypho-scoliosis in the thoracic region
Figure 4D. Human spine showing severe scoliosis with crowding of ribs on concave side of curvature

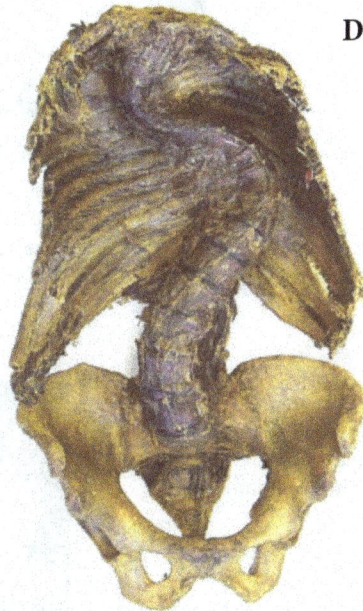

VERTEBRAE

Cervical vertebrae

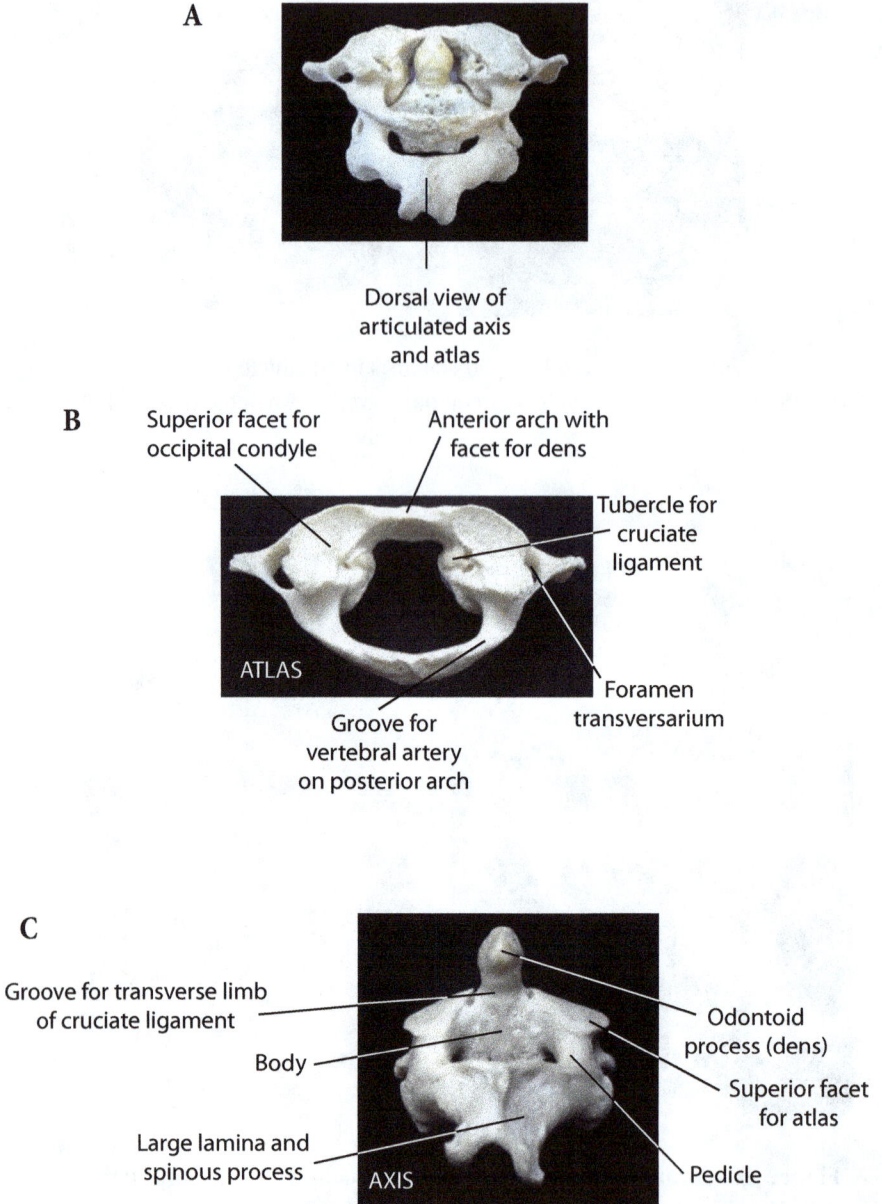

A

Dorsal view of
articulated axis
and atlas

B

Superior facet for
occipital condyle

Anterior arch with
facet for dens

Tubercle for
cruciate
ligament

ATLAS

Groove for
vertebral artery
on posterior arch

Foramen
transversarium

C

Groove for transverse limb
of cruciate ligament

Body

Large lamina and
spinous process

AXIS

Odontoid
process (dens)

Superior facet
for atlas

Pedicle

Figure 5. Atypical cervical vertebrae
(A) Atlas (C1) and axis (C2)
(B) Atlas (C1); (C) axis (C2)

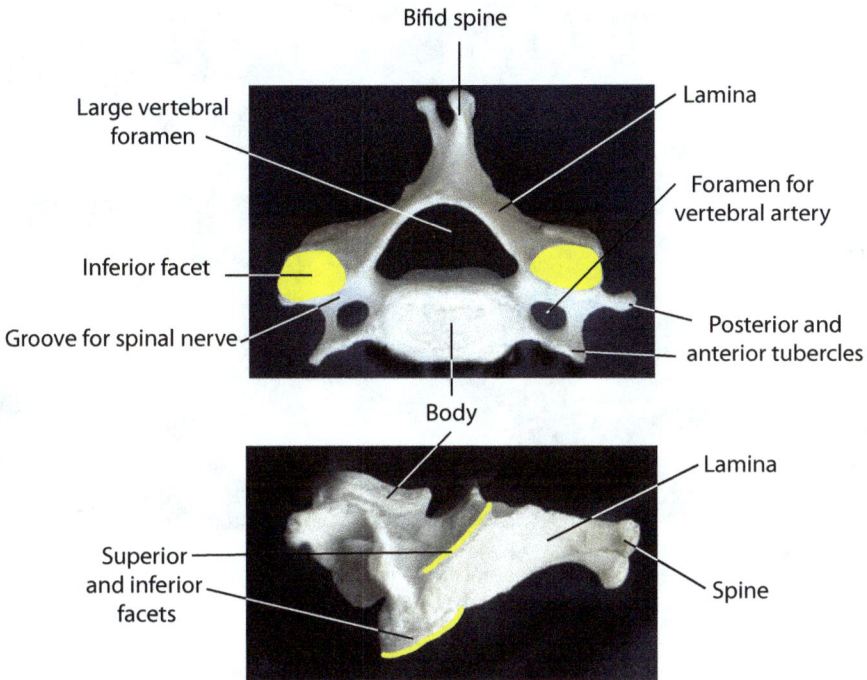

Figure 6. Typical cervical vertebrae

The typical cervical vertebra (Figure 6) has a small spine and body but a comparatively large vertebral (spinal) foramen to allow for the wide range of movements characteristic of the region and to accommodate the cervical enlargement of the cord which gives origin to the cervical and brachial plexuses. The oblique orientation of the articular facets (Figure 8) shows how movements in several planes are possible. A unique feature is the foramen in the transverse process (Figure 6), which transmits the vertebral artery (and vein) and provides, through the vertebro-basilar system, the blood supply to vital parts of the brain, including visual cortex, brain stem, cerebellum and upper spinal cord. The atlas (C1) and axis (C2) vertebrae (Figure 5) are much larger and specially adapted to support the skull and provide articulation with the skull allowing the head a wide range of movement. The pivot joint between the odontoid process of the axis and the anterior arch of the atlas is a critical articulation, disruption of which can lead to catastrophic results. The large spine of the axis provides attachment for powerful antigravity neck muscles to keep the neck upright.

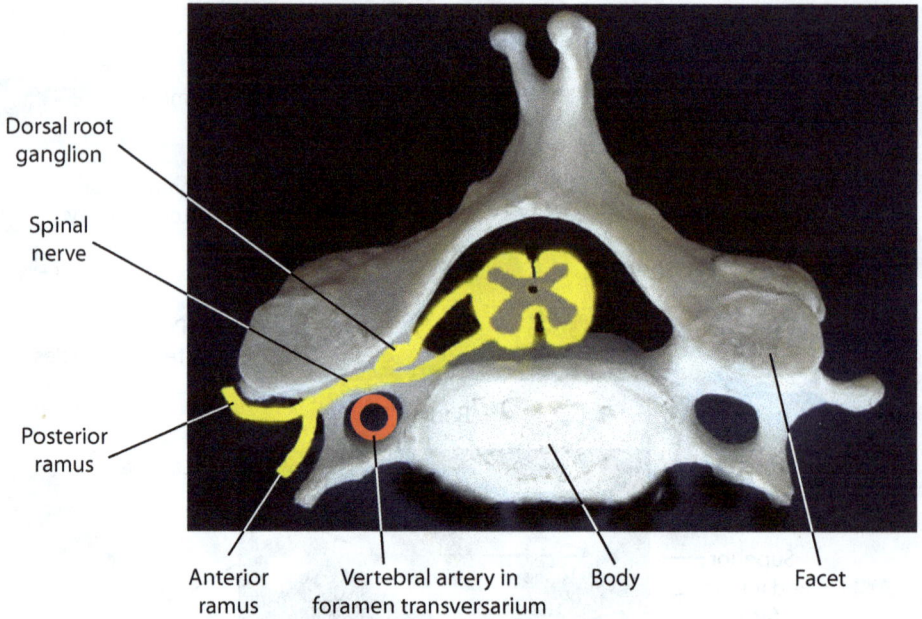

Figure 7. The spinal cord, spinal nerve and vertebral artery in relation to a cervical vertebra

The spinal nerve and dorsal root ganglion (Figure 7) lie in the intervertebral foramen, close to the intervertebral disc and facet (zygapophyseal) joints where the nerve is vulnerable to encroachment. The vertebral artery ascends the neck through the foramina transversaria in the transverse processes. It also is vulnerable to compression by disc prolapse and osteophytes associated with facet joints degeneration.

Stability of the cervical spine (excluding the specialised C1 and 2 vertebrae) depends on two bony columns, anterior and posterior, which can be defined in the articulated spine. The anterior column (centrum element) comprises the vertebral bodies and intervertebral discs linked by anterior and posterior longitudinal ligaments. The posterior column (neural-arch element) comprises the pedicles, transverse processes, laminae and ligamenta flava, also the spinous processes with the interspinous, and supraspinous ligaments. Disruption of either or both of these columns results in spinal instability.

Odontoid process (dens) of the axis

Groove for vertebral artery
on posterior arch of atlas

Spine of axis

Facet joints

C6 spine

Intervertebral disc

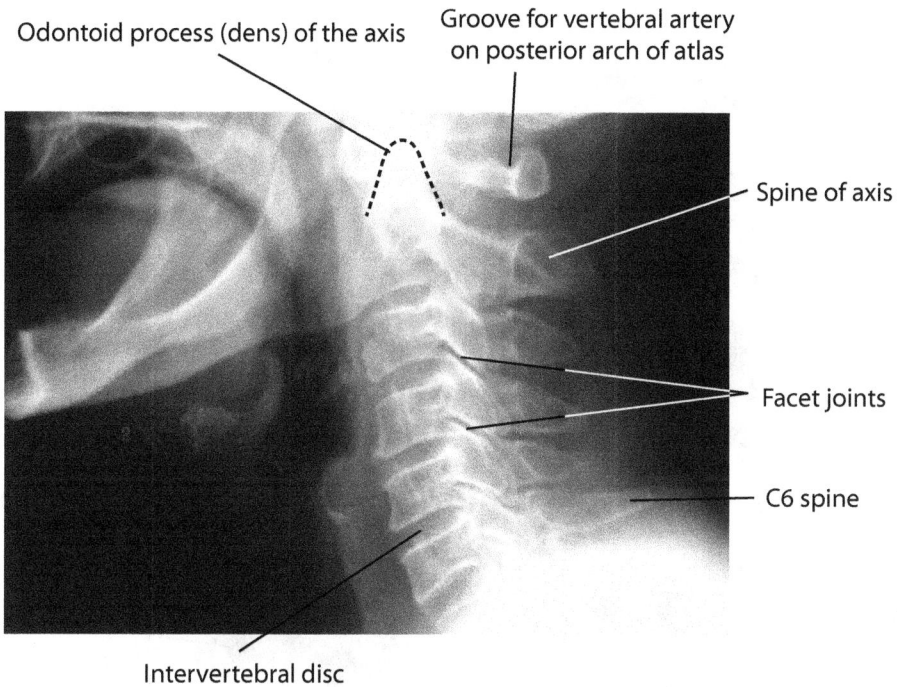

Figure 8. Lateral x- radiograph of cervical spine

Thoracic vertebrae

Thoracic vertebrae are larger than the cervical and typically have long spinous processes (Figure 9), which overlap each other thereby restricting movement particularly in the mid-thoracic region. Characteristically they articulate with ribs and this further restricts movement especially in a coronal plane. Since there is no thoracic enlargement of the spinal cord the spinal canal is relatively small. Of all the movements possible in this part of the spine the direction of the articular facets indicates that rotation is the most free.

Osteochondritis of growth endplates of the vertebral bodies (Schuermann's disease) (Figure 9a) occurs in younger ages especially in the thoracic spine and is associated with pain and thoracic kyphosis. Costo-vertebral joints may be involved in stress, osteo-arthritis and ankylosing spondylitis causing pain.

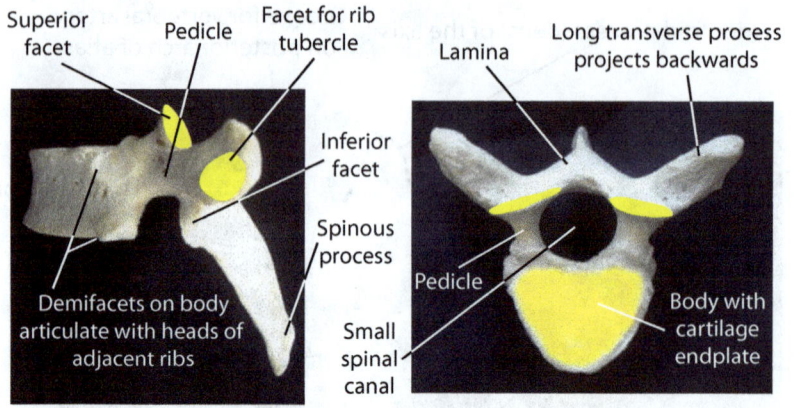

RIB ARTICULATIONS WITH VERTEBRAE

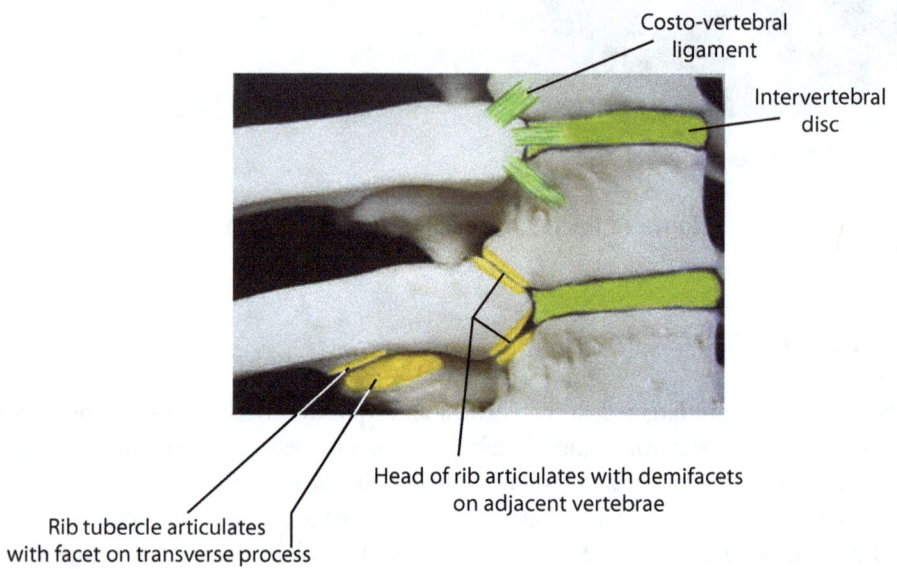

Figure 9. Thoracic vertebrae and articulation with ribs

In a study of the capsules of human costo-transverse joints, Dendrick *et al.* (2011) detected somatic and autonomic neuropeptides of the type associated with pain mediation (e.g. substance P) and suggest these joints can be a source of thoracic pain. Young *et al.* (2008) described local referral of pain from costo-transverse joints to (the region of thoracic) paraspinal muscles. Erwini *et al.* (2000) described referral of pain from costo-vertebral joints to a similar site, namely the region of paraspinal muscles.

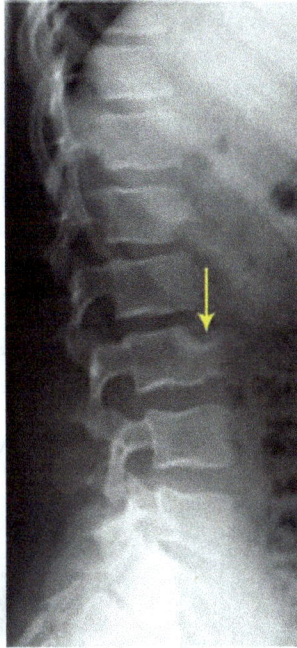

Figure 9a. Lateral X-radiograph of the lower spine indicating Schuermann's disease. The arrow shows typical scalloping erosion of the superior endplate of the L3 vertebra

PROBLEM No. 1

A 24 year old male Olympic sweep rower who normally competes in a four man boat complains of low intensity central mid thoracic pain that comes on after approximately 90 minutes and gradually worsens throughout the rest of a typical three hour rowing training session. The problem arose approximately four weeks ago and coincided with an increase in the number and intensity of on-water rowing sessions. It is not intense enough to stop him rowing however he feels it is beginning to hamper his stroke power and it now comes on earlier and is more intense by the end of the session. The pain is described as a deep ache that is at worst rated as 6 out of 10 on a visual analogue scale (0 being no pain and 10, the worst imaginable pain). He also has pain radiating to his left side to the mid-axillary line along the line of the 7th rib. He rows with the oar on the right side. The rower is otherwise well although earlier in the year he did suffer a period of unexplained underperformance and fatigue. Blood tests at the time were normal apart from a low Vitamin D level.

i)   List at least five structures that could be the source of the discomfort?
ii)   What is the likely mechanism of injury?
iii)   Which dermatome (Figure 49) is associated with the pattern of pain radiation?
iv)   What might be the potential significance of a low Vitamin D level?
v)   What costal pathology is common in rowers that might result in the described pattern of pain?
vi)   What pattern of spinal curvature might you see expect to see in this athlete?
vii)   How might symptoms of forearm and hand pain, coldness and abnormally high perspiration be associated with this problem?

Lumbar vertebrae

The lumbar vertebrae are the largest and most sturdy of all. This reflects their role in supporting the considerable weight of the head, neck and trunk. The vertebral bodies are large, and the spinous processes are large and prominent (Figure 10) giving attachment to the strong erector spinae group of antigravity muscles. Much of the body is cancellous trabeculated bone. The trabeculae are not arranged randomly, some are vertical to resist vertical compression and others are transverse (Figure 11) acting as tie-beams between them to give added support to the vertical group.

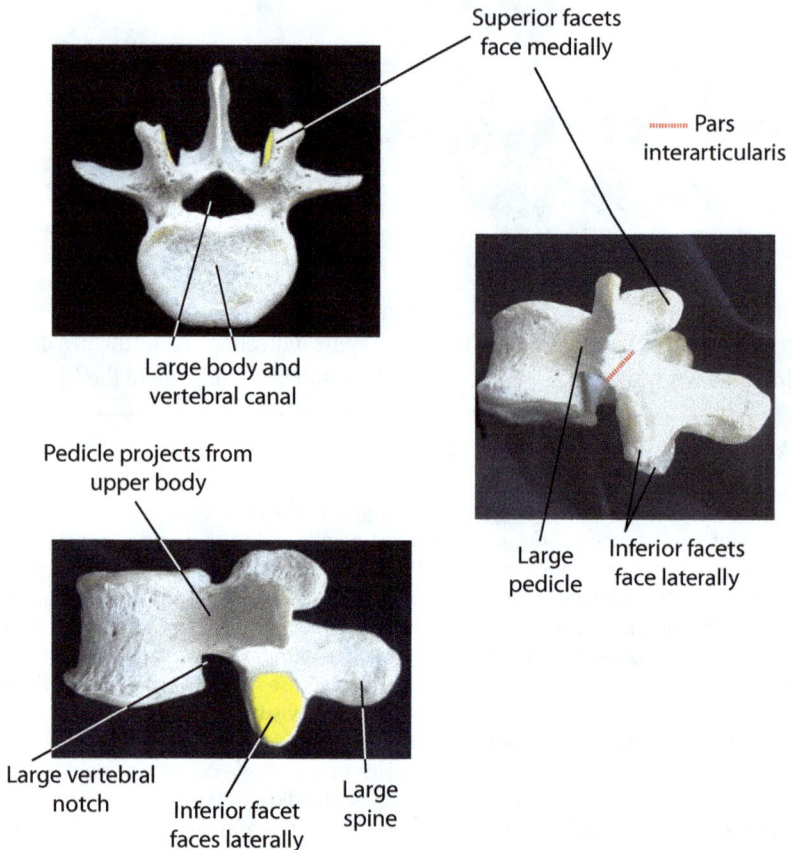

Figure 10. Lumbar vertebrae

In osteopenia and osteoporosis bone tissue decreases due to loss of both inorganic and organic matrix with concomitant disruption and disappearance of trabeculae and weakening of the bone. Older athletes and those susceptible to the female athlete triad of low energy availability (with or without eating disorders), amenorrhea and osteoporosis may be at risk of vertebral bone stress injury (Nattiv, *et al.*, 2007). In severe cases of reduced bone density the end-result may be collapse of the vertebral body.

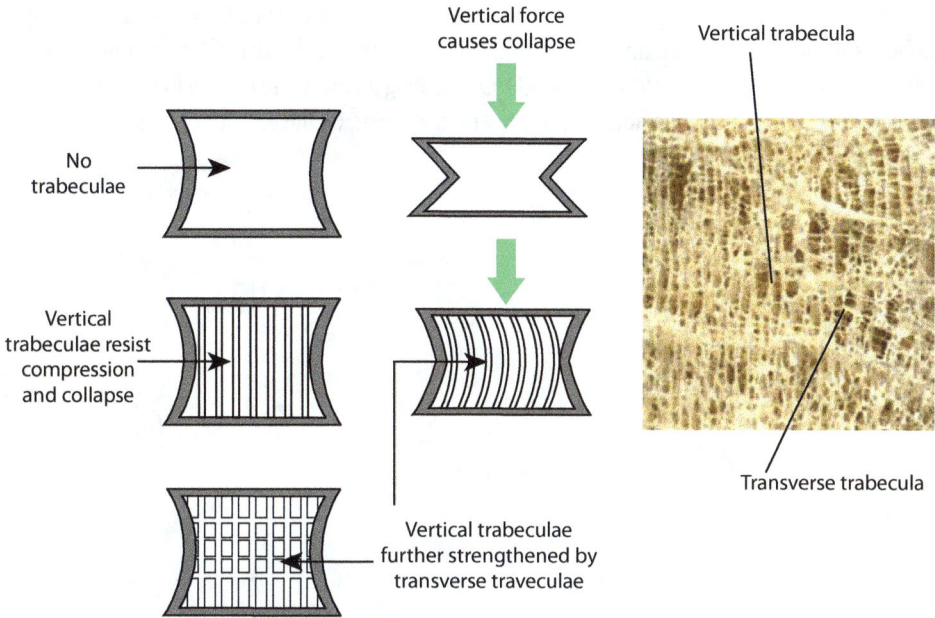

Figure 11. Bony architecture of vertebral body

Important features of lumbar vertebrae are:

- The attachment of the pedicles to the upper half of the body (Figures 10 & 12), leaving the lower half free to form with the adjacent vertebra a large intervertebral foramen for emergence of the spinal nerve so that it lies clear of the adjacent intervertebral disc
- The spinal canal is large and lodges the cauda equina
- In mature adults narrowing of the spinal canal may impinge on the cord causing neurological claudication with weakness of the legs and pain on exercise
- The pars interarticularis which is the region between the upper and lower articular processes and facets (Figure 10) may be the site of spondylolysis

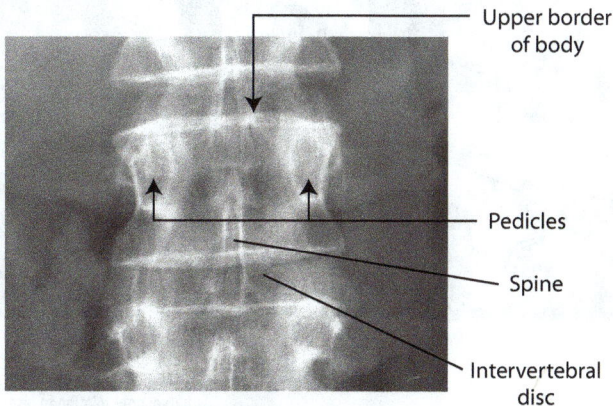

Figure 12. Antero-Posterior X-radiograph of the lumbar spine

In the upright posture the angle subtended between the upper border of L1 vertebra and the upper surface of the sacrum is approximately 70° and between the upper border of the sacrum and lower border of L5 the angle is about 16° (Figure 13). On bending forwards the normal lordosis disappears and body weight produces dual forces, compressive and shear, on the intervertebral joints.

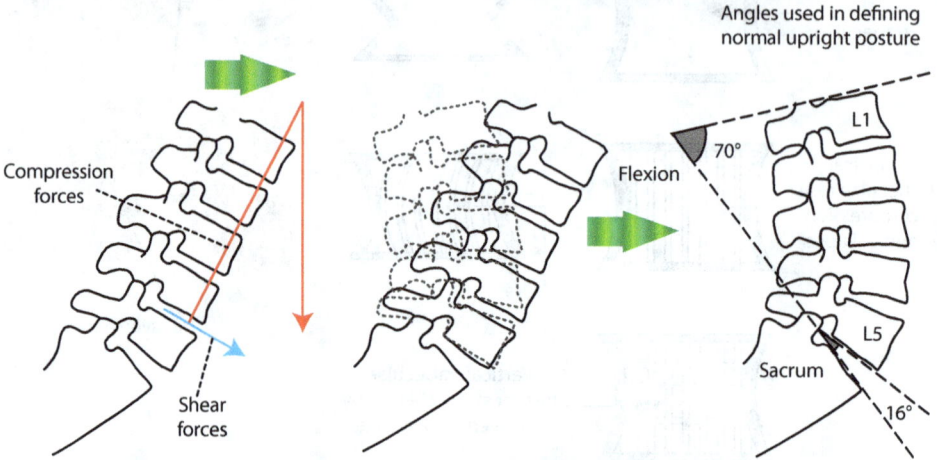

Figure 13. Forces associated with movement of the lumbar spine

The intervertebral foramen is one of the most important patho-anatomical locations in the spine especially in the cervical and lumbar regions. A number of structures form its boundaries including the intervertebral disc and the facet (zygapophyseal) joint (Figure 14) and also the ligamentum flavum (Figure 23). These are significant since they may cause encroachment and compression of emerging roots of a spinal nerve. This may result from disc prolapse or arthritic changes in the synovial facet joint. Hypertrophy of the ligamentum flavum has been proposed as a potential cause of posterior thigh and calf pain and muscle strains in mature athletes (Orchard, *et al.*, 2004).

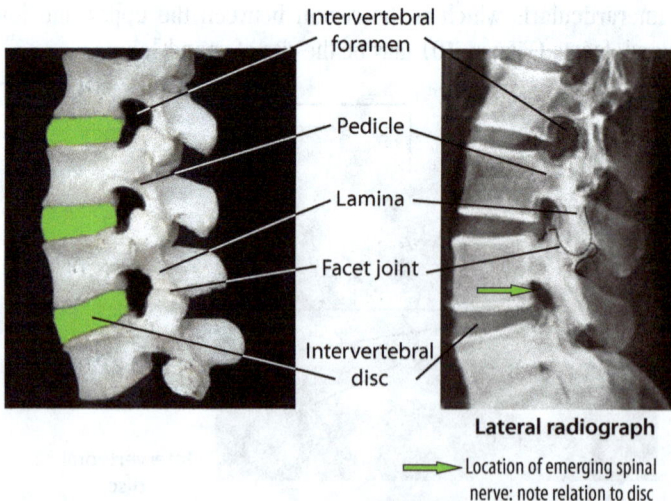

Figure 14. The intervertebral foramen and its boundaries

The sacrum is the terminal part of the spinal column consisting of five fused sacral vertebrae. It forms the major articulation between the column and the pelvic girdle at the sacroiliac joints. The sacral canal contains the lower part of the dural sac together with the sacral and coccygeal nerves. The nerves emerge as ventral and dorsal rami through conspicuous foramina on the front and back of the sacrum (Figure 15). The coccyx, varies considerably in size and mobility, and articulates with the restricted distal end of the sacrum.

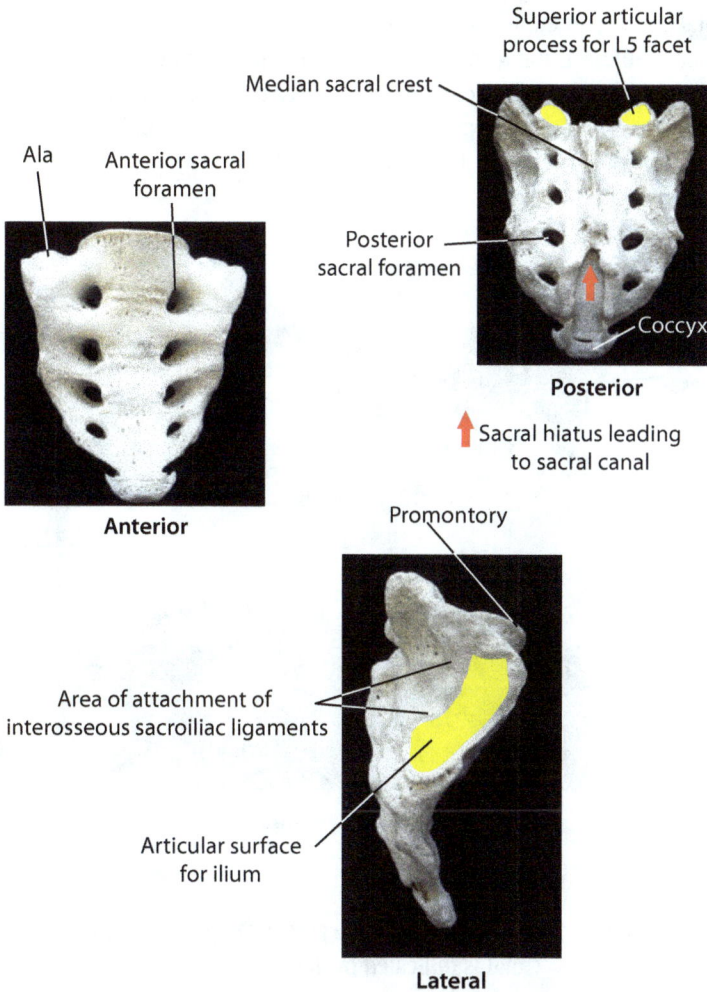

Figure 15. The sacrum and coccyx

Spondylolysis and Spondylolisthesis

Spondylolysis (Figure 16) is any spinal lesion of a degenerative nature which may be dysplastic (developmental) or due to cumulative micro-trauma to the posterior bony elements or facet joints. Cumulative micro-trauma to the pedicles and partes interarticulares of the lower lumbar spine results in a high incidence of acute stress fracture injury in athletes involved in sports requiring repeated lumbar extension such as swimming, gymnastics, baseball pitching and fast bowling in cricket (Figures 17 & 18).

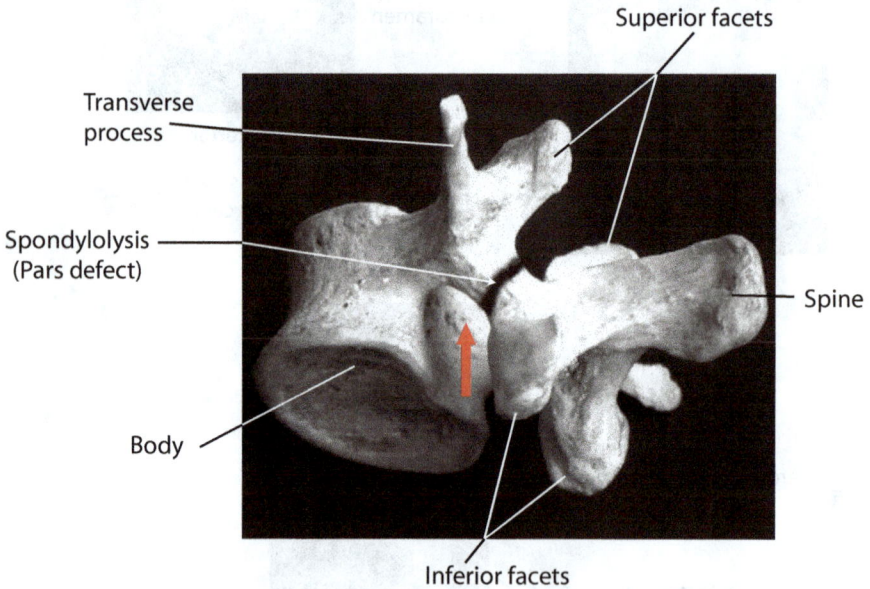

Figure 16. Spondylolysis indicated by black line across the pars interarticularis. The spinal canal is indicated by the red arrow

Acute pedicle bone stress reaction

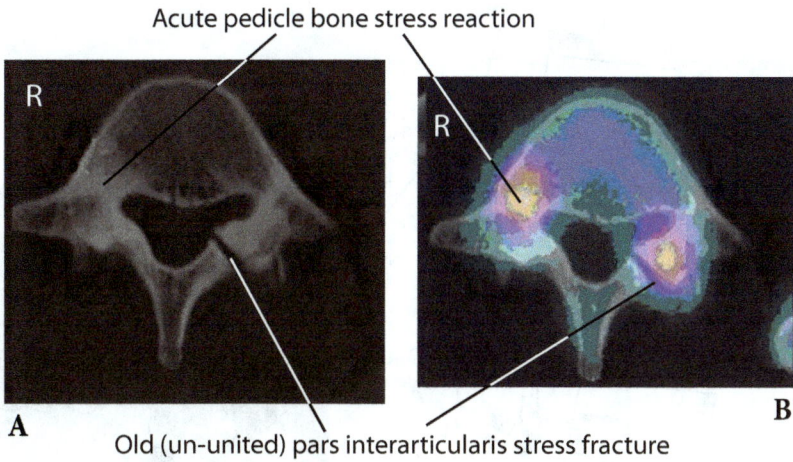

A   B

Old (un-united) pars interarticularis stress fracture

Figure 17. A) Axial CT showing a left un-united pars interarticularis stress fracture with adjacent acute fracture fragments, and thickening of the right pedicle **B)** superimposed single photon emission CT (SPECT) diagnostic scan with colours indicating areas of bone stress reaction in the left pars and right pedicle

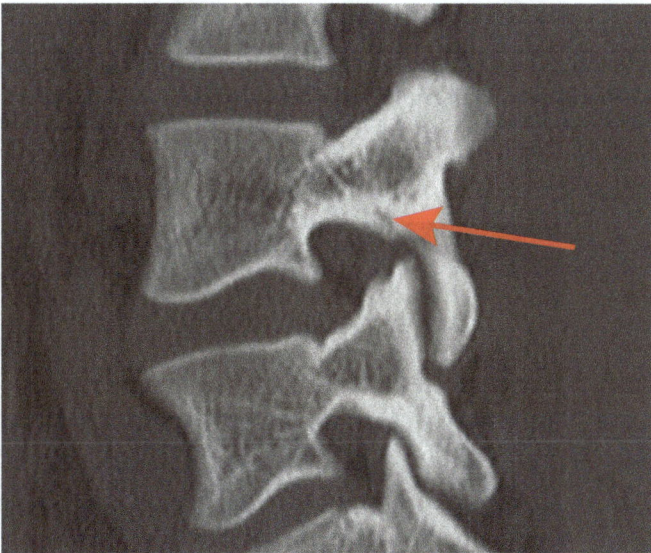

Figure 18. Sagittal CT scan of a partial stress fracture of the L4 pedicle in a cricket fast bowler

Complete bilateral stress fracture may lead to separation (spondylolysis) between the posterior neural arch element of the vertebra (spine, laminae and inferior articular processes) and the anterior centrum area (body, transverse process and superior articular process). Anterior slippage of these bony elements lying anterior to the fractures is termed spondylolysthesis (Figure 19) with effects on the cauda equina, such as pain in the distribution of L4 or L5 spinal nerve. In asymmetrical sports such as cricket, baseball and tennis, chronic stress is identifiable by unilateral thickening and sclerosis of the posterior bony elements (Figure 20) (Ranson, *et al.*, 2005).

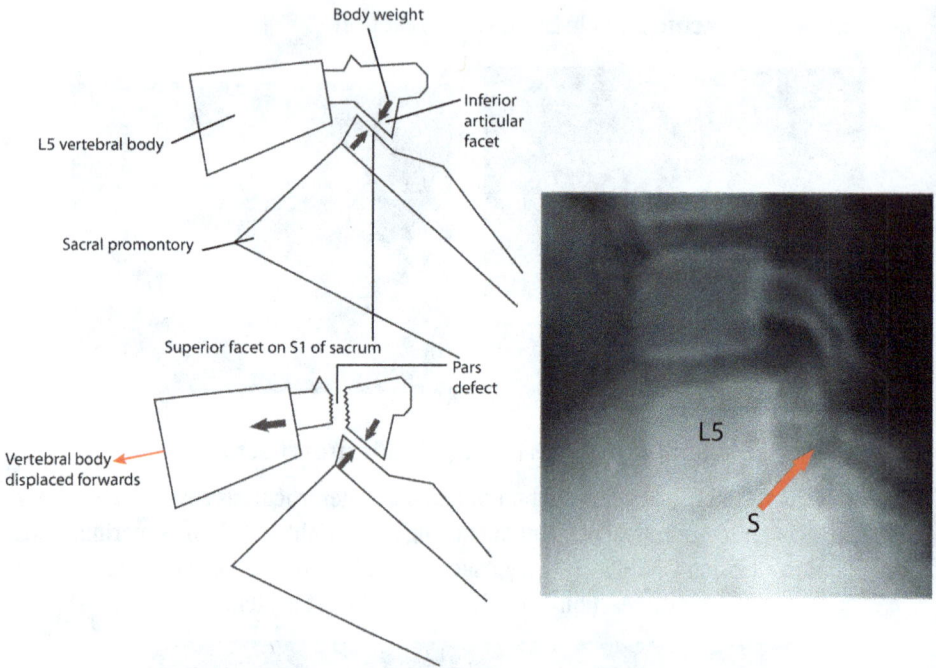

Figure19. Spondylolisthesis – anterior slip of the L5 vertebral body and pedicle due to bilateral disruption of the partes interarticulares (red arrow)

(By permission from Rockwater Inc. Mitchell GAG (1934) The lumbo-sacral junction *J.Bone Joint Surg A.* **16** 233-254 Figures 5 and 14)

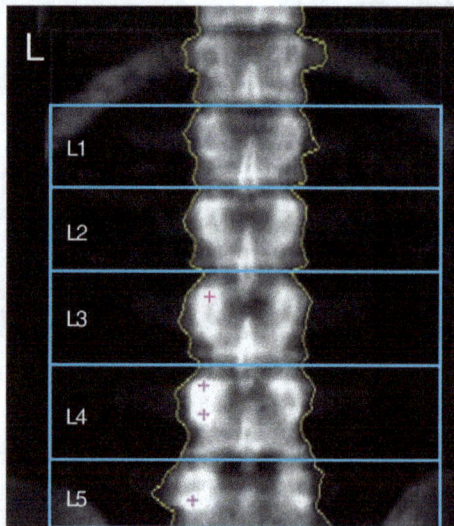

Figure 20. Dual Energy X-ray Absorbiometry (DEXA) scan showing unilateral left sided thickening and sclerosis of the L3, 4 and 5 posterior bony elements (red crosses) due to the repetitive stress of left lumbar side-flexion during fast bowling in cricket

PROBLEM No. 2

A 25 year old female Olympic javelin thrower is complaining of left sided lower back pain that is preventing her from throwing. She is a right arm thrower. She initially noticed mild discomfort (2/10 on a visual analogue pain scale) localised to the L4 region of her left lower back two months ago that was only present during throwing sessions. At that stage she had no back discomfort with any other training or activities of daily living (ADL). Resting from throwing for 7-10 days would ease the pain at the next throwing session but it would return within one or two further sessions.

Over the last four weeks the discomfort gradually worsened so that now it is 8/10, preventing her from throwing maximally. Most ADL and training activities remain pain free apart from when she bends fully backwards during strength training activities.

There is no pain radiation to the buttock or lower limb. No pain with coughing or sneezing. No symptoms of neurological dysfunction e.g. no weakness or numbness in the trunk, buttocks or lower limbs.

i)   What structures could possibly be involved?
ii)   What is the likely mechanism of injury?
iii) In order of likelihood, what are three possible diagnoses?
iv)   Which features of the history might lead you to exclude intervertebral disc injury as one of the likely diagnoses?
v)   Which features of the history might lead you to include bone injury as one of the likely diagnoses?
vi)   What positive findings would you expect on physical examination?
vii) What other sporting activities involve the type of extreme asymmetrical spinal movement that may produce similar unilateral lower back injuries?
viii) Which radiological investigations might be appropriate?

Spinal Joints

Types of joints: The joints of the spine can be classified into three types. They can be summarised as the "3 Ss" :

- Syndesmoses (fibrous joints) comprising the inter-transverse, inter-spinous and supra-spinous, anterior and posterior longitudinal ligaments
- Synovial joints between the articular facets (zygapophyseal)
- Symphysis (secondary cartilaginous) comprising the intervertebral discs between the vertebral bodies

Syndesmoses

Between adjacent vertebrae short fibrous ligaments connect the transverse and spinous processes. They are strong but if stretched or torn may be a cause of lower back pain. The anterior and posterior longitudinal fibrous ligaments are much more extensive, attaching to the vertebral bodies and intervertebral discs as they traverse the whole length of the spine (Figure 21). The anterior ligament is broad and prevents any forward prolapse of intervertebral discs. The posterior ligament is more narrow with a denticulate appearance (Figure 22). It is not sufficiently wide to always prevent central disc prolapse against the spinal cord. More commonly it does permit postero-lateral prolapse towards the intervertebral foramen and spinal nerve.

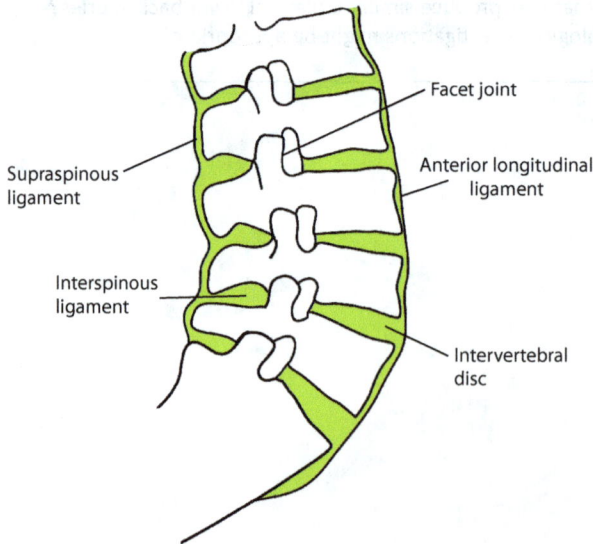

Figure 21. Lateral view of fibrous and facet joints

Intervertebral disc

Pedicles cut to expose
vertebral bodies

Transverse process

Inter-transverse
ligaments

Posterior longitudinal ligament on
dorsum of vertebral bodies

Broad anterior longitudinal
ligament adheres to discs

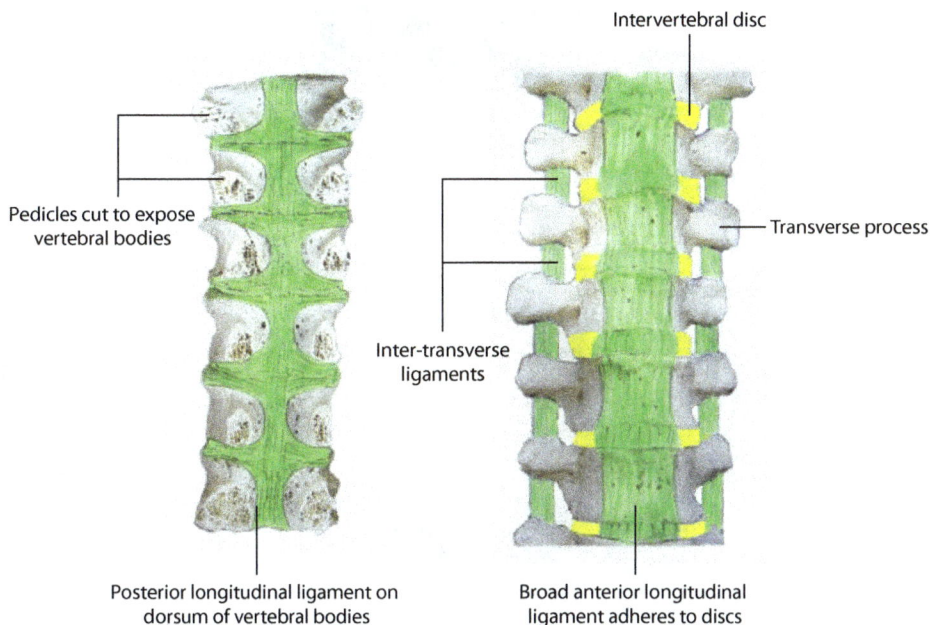

Figure 22. Posterior and anterior longitudinal ligaments.
The inter-transverse ligaments are also shown

The laminae of adjacent vertebral arches are connected by elastic ligamenta flava (Figures 23 & 24). These help to restore and maintain the upright posture. With sudden hyperextension of the spine as occurs in whiplash injuries of the spine the ligamenta flava may herniate into the spinal canal causing spinal nerve or cord compression.

In the cervical vertebrae the large ligamentum nuchae (Figures 24 & 25), composed of elastic fibres surmounts the spinous processes and extends upwards onto the external occipital crest as far as the external occipital protuberance. It has a posterior free margin to which the trapezius muscles and deep investing fascia of the neck are attached.

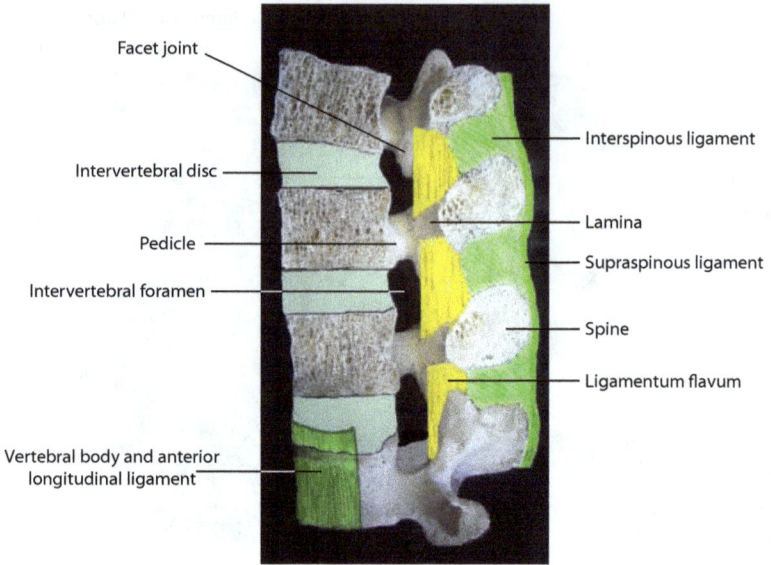

Figure 23. Median sagittal section of lumbar spine to view intervertebral foramina from within spinal canal. The ligamentum flavum is in close relation to the intervertebral foramen

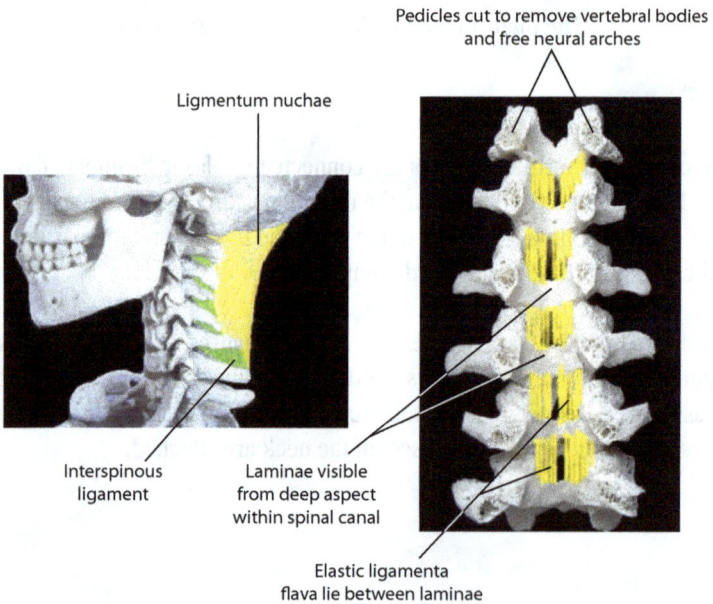

Figure 24. The ligamentum nuchae and ligamenta flava. The ligamenta flava are viewed as seen from inside the spinal canal

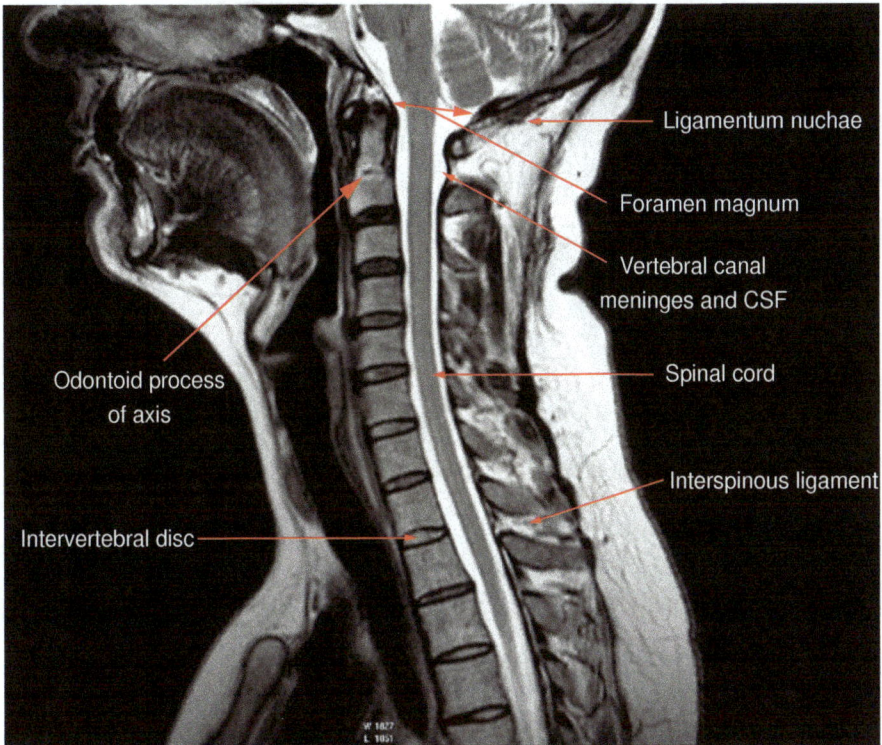

Figure 25. Median sagittal MRI scan of the cervical spine

Synovial joints

These joints, also called zygapophyseal, lie between adjacent articular facets and have the same structure as synovial joints elsewhere in the body. The articular surfaces which are covered by hyaline cartilage are separated by a narrow cavity (Figures 26a, b & c) and enclosed by a fibrous capsule (Figure 26a). Non-articular surfaces and the interior of the capsule are lined by synovial membrane which produces a small amount of synovial fluid to lubricate the articular cartilage (Figures 27a & b). Being synovial joints they may be involved in any of the types of arthritis affecting synovial joints, causing pain and stiffness also swelling which may impinge on adjacent nerves including spinal nerves emerging through intervertebral foramina and dorsal rami. The direction in which articular facets face determines the direction of movement of particular regions of the spine. Thus in the cervical region they allow wide ranges of movement, forward and lateral flexion, extension and rotation. In the thoracic region, especially mid-thoracic, they allow rotation but otherwise movements are considerably restricted by the presence of ribs. In the lumbar region flexion and extension are free but other movements especially rotation are much restricted.

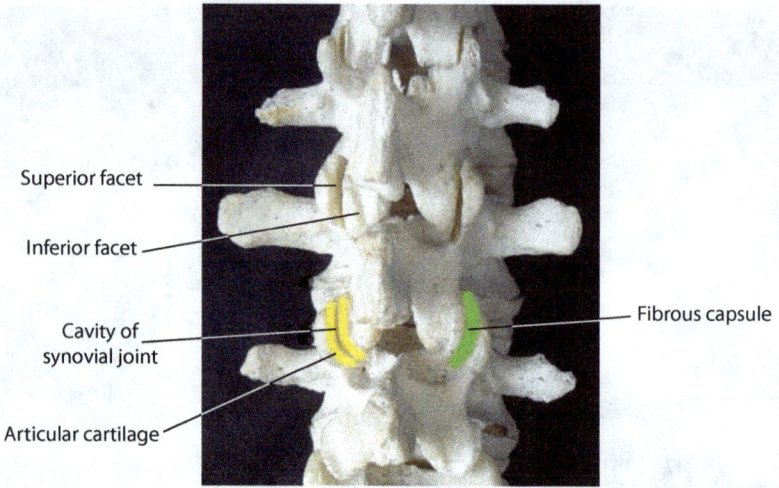

Figure 26a. Dorsal view of synovial lumbar vertebral facet (zygapophysial) joints

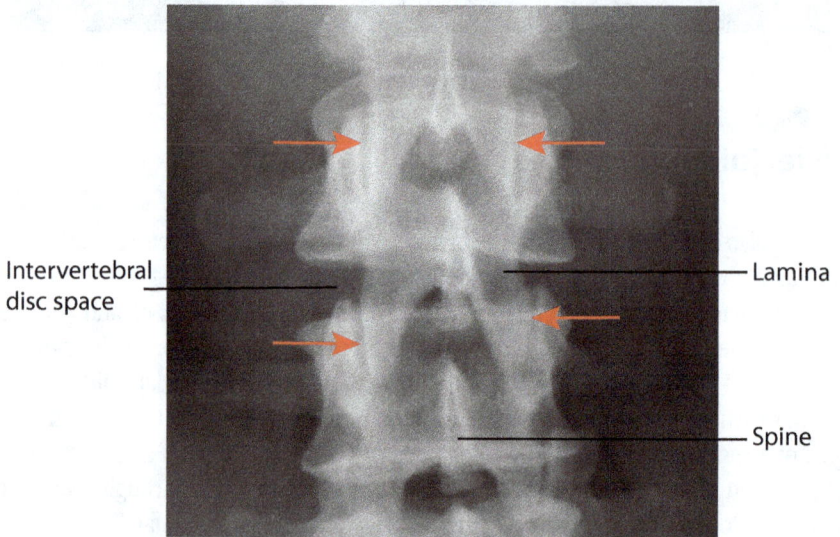

Figure 26b. Antero-posterior X-radiograph of lumbar spine. Facet joints are labeled with red arrows

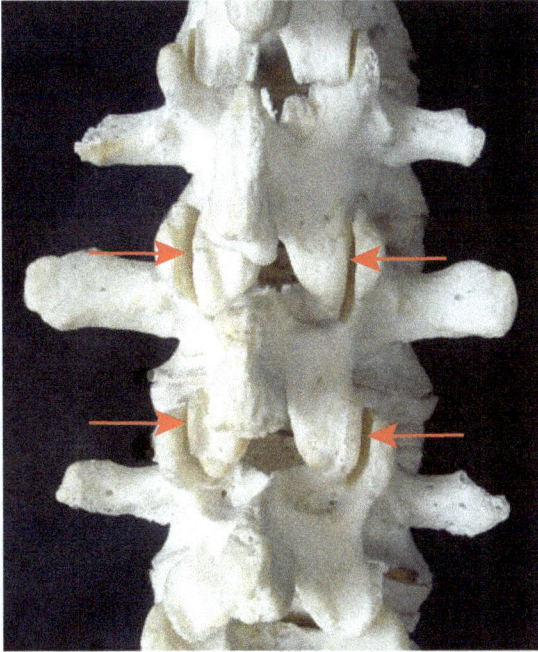

Figure 26c. Dorsal view of facet joints which are labeled with red arrows

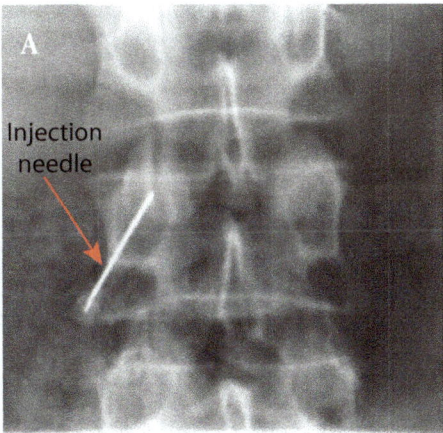

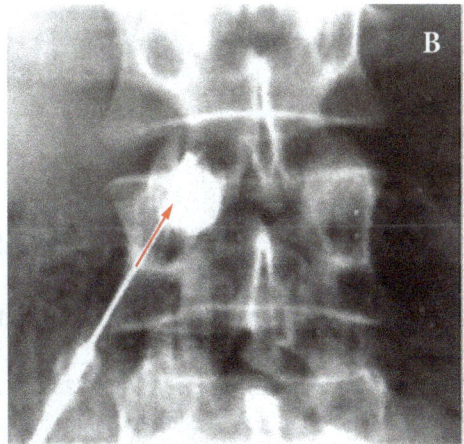

Figure 27. a) Fluoroscopy of needle insertion into lumbar facet joint b) opaque medium indicating injected fluid within the joint (red arrow)

Symphysis joints

These comprise the intervertebral discs and are associated with significant morbidity in the spine. They account for nearly 25% of the total length of the spine excluding the sacrum and vary in thickness according to the region, being thickest in the lumbar spine, less thick in the cervical and thinnest in the thoracic area (Figure 28). Thickness is directly related to the amount of weight bearing and of movement. It is also related to disc prolapse which is most common in the lumbar region, moderately common in the cervical region and least common in the thoracic spine.

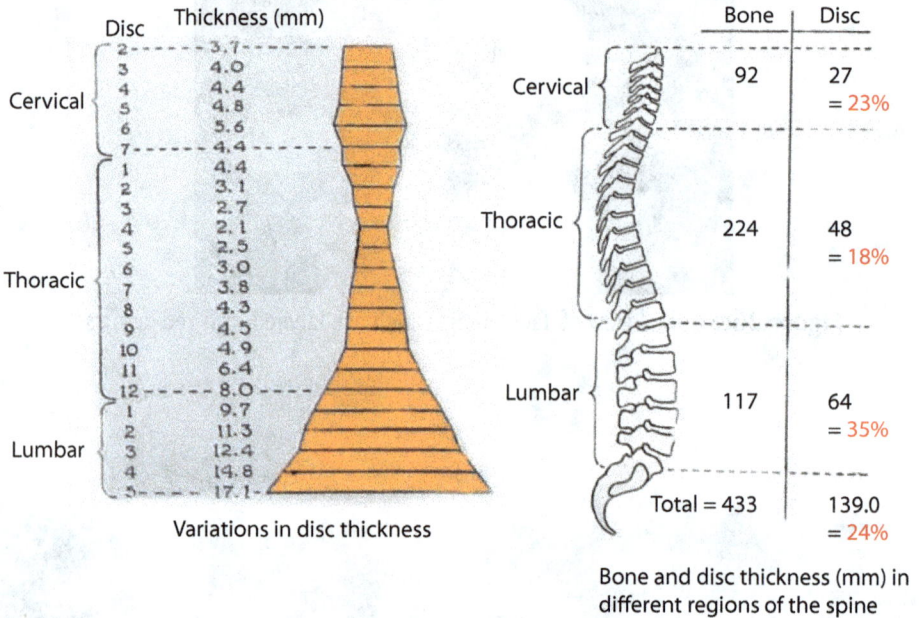

Disc	Thickness (mm)
Cervical 2	3.7
3	4.0
4	4.4
5	4.8
6	5.6
7	4.4
Thoracic 1	4.4
2	3.1
3	2.7
4	2.1
5	2.5
6	3.0
7	3.8
8	4.3
9	4.5
10	4.9
11	6.4
12	8.0
Lumbar 1	9.7
2	11.3
3	12.4
4	14.8
5	17.1

Variations in disc thickness

	Bone	Disc
Cervical	92	27 = 23%
Thoracic	224	48 = 18%
Lumbar	117	64 = 35%
Total = 433		139.0 = 24%

Bone and disc thickness (mm) in different regions of the spine

Figure 28. Regional variations in thickness of intervertebral discs

Structure: Each disc has an outer lamellated fibrous zone, the annulus fibrosus, and an inner more amorphous gelatinous zone, the nucleus pulposus which is usually located slightly posterior to the centre of the disc. The boundary between the two zones is indistinct. The annulus contains collagen fibres which have a regular orientation in each layer, with each layer lying diagonally opposed to the adjacent layer (Figure 29). This alternating pattern in direction is repeated throughout the lamellae in the annulus.

Individual lamellae are linked by radially orientated translamellar fibres that form bridges between the lamellae (Figure 30). These bridges help to stabilise the lamellae and limit slip between lamellae (Schollum, *et al.*, 2009), which accompanies flexion, extension and torsion of the spine. The ground substance is composed of mucopolysaccharides whose function is to bind water in the annulus and especially in the nucleus pulposus. This provides the disc with an important physical property making it turgid like a well-inflated balloon and producing a remarkably high intrinsic pressure. Thus in vivo measurements by Wilke *et al.*,(1999) of a normal lumbar disc with the subject lying recumbent found pressures of MPa 0.10 -0.11 (14.5 – 17.5 psi). Activities such as forward flexion of the trunk and the carrying of a heavy weight resulted in dramatic rises in pressure . These pressures were 1.10MPa (160psi) during forward flexion and 2.3MPa (333psi) when carrying a 20kg load whilst bending (Wilke, *et al.*, 1999). In the living spine, whether standing or sitting, the movement of flexion greatly increases intra-disc pressure.

These structural features are the basis of three important functions of discs:

- Shock-absorption allowing vertical forces to be moderated
- Transmission of forces along the spinal column from vertebra to vertebra
- Allowing movement but resisting torsion (twisting movements)

Nucleus pulposus

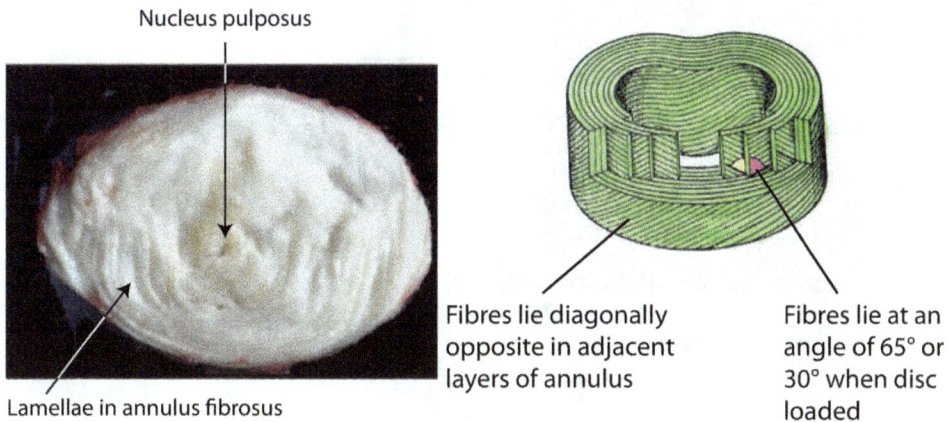

Lamellae in annulus fibrosus

Fibres lie diagonally opposite in adjacent layers of annulus

Fibres lie at an angle of 65° or 30° when disc loaded

Figure 29. Structure of an intervertebral disc

Vertical force applied to the disc causes pressure to increase in the nucleus pulposus. This is transmitted outwards causing the annulus fibres to stretch and then recoil and brace against the nucleus. Being braced, fibres of the annulus which are embedded in the cartilage endplate of the vertebra are able to transmit force between adjacent vertebrae (Figure 31).

An important factor influencing pressure effects on intervertebral discs and vertebral bodies is the supporting role of intra-abdominal pressure provided by the 'thoraco-abdominal balloon' when lifting. Contraction of muscles of the anterior abdominal wall, the diaphragm and the pelvic floor raises intra-abdominal pressure which is equivalent to inflating a balloon in front

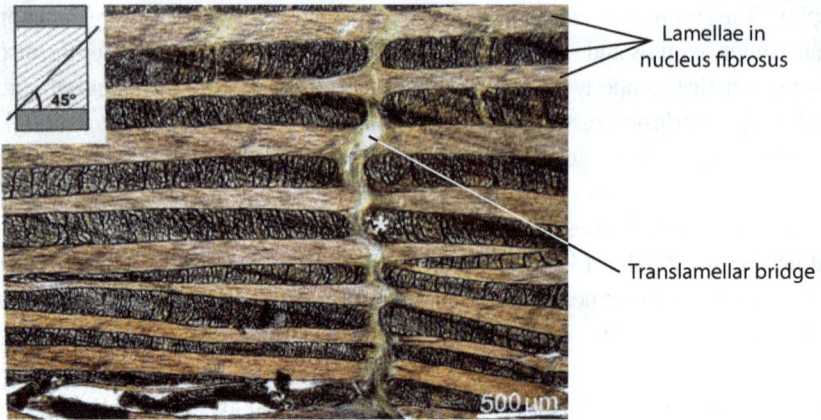

Figure 30. Translamellar bridges in nucleus fibrosus
(reproduced with permission from Schollum ML, Roberton PA and Broom ND A
microstructural investigation of intervertebral disc lamellar connectivity: detailed analysis of
the translamellar bridges (2009) *J. Anat.* **214** 805-816 Figure 2 Wiley-Blackwell)

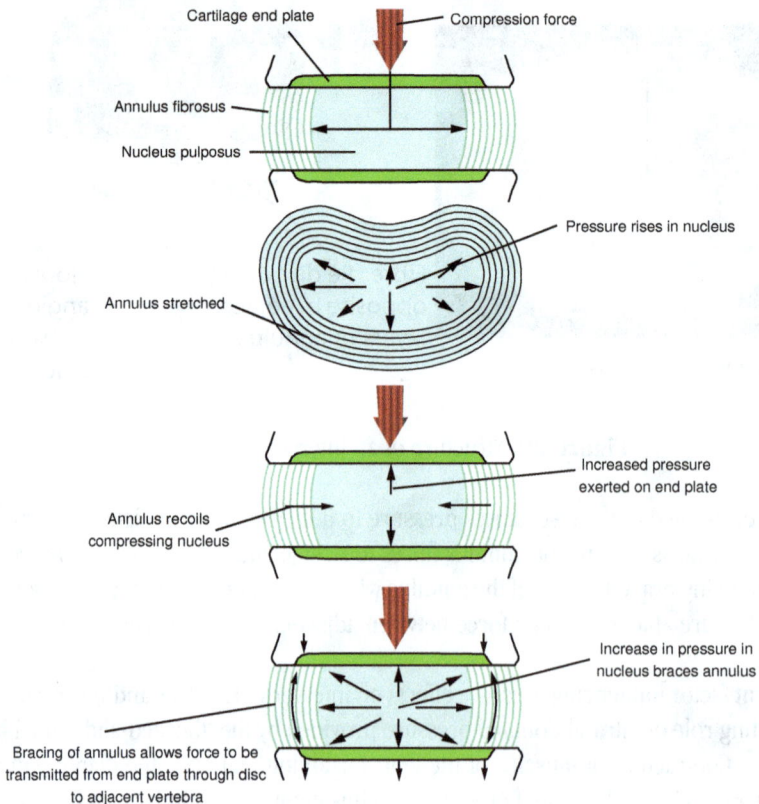

Figure 31. Functional anatomy of the intervertebral disc

of the vertebral column which acts as a splint. This may be critical when lifting heavy weights. Without it, weights which could normally be lifted would cause disc and vertebral collapse (Figure 32).

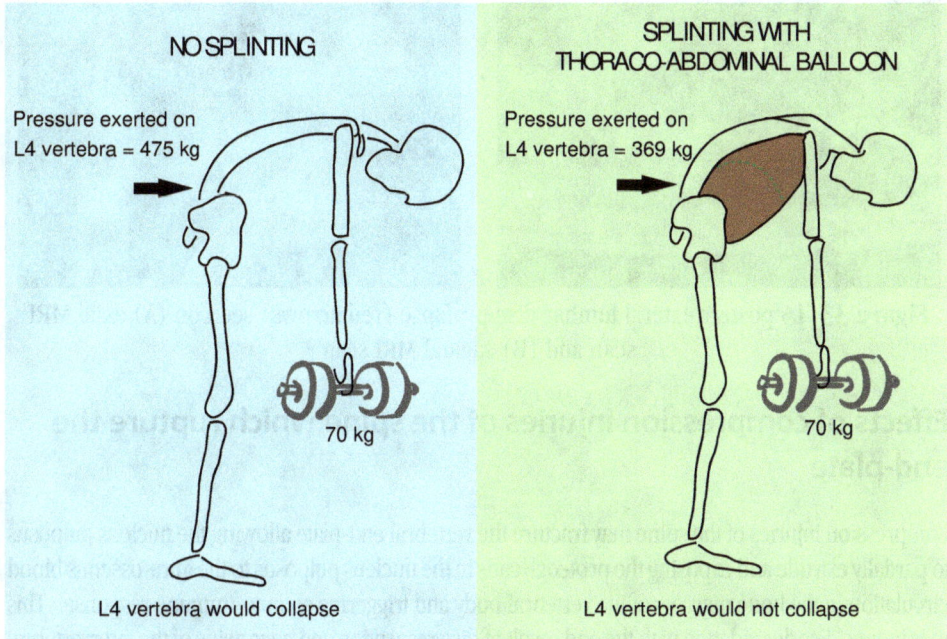

Figure 32. The splinting effect of intra-abdominal pressure on the spine

Disc collapse and herniation

The normal disc holds a large amount of water which is bound to mucopolysaccharide in the gelatinous matrix. As age increases, due to depolymerisation of the mucopolysaccharide, the amount of water bound in the matrix decreases causing the disc to dry and collagen fibres in the annulus to crack. The nucleus pulposus herniates through the cracks towards the disc surface like toothpaste extruding from its tube.

Prolapse may occur in one of three directions:

- Postero-laterally with impingement on a spinal nerve (Figures 33 & 45)
- Posteriorly with impingement on the spinal cord or cauda equina (Figures 34 & 45)
- Superiorly or inferiorly through the endplate into the trabeculated bone of an adjacent vertebral body forming a 'Schmorl's body' with narrowing of the disc space

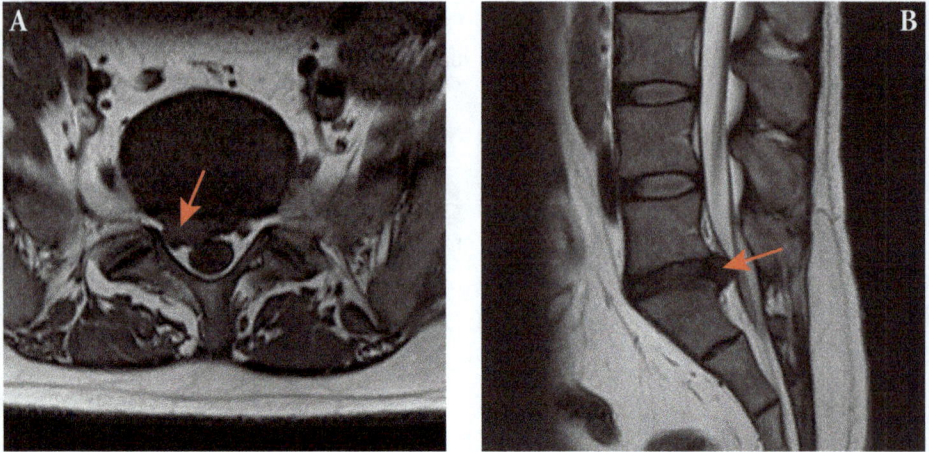

Figure 33. L5 postero-lateral lumbar disc prolapse (red arrows) seen on (A) axial MRI scan and (B) sagittal MRI scan

Effects of compression injuries of the spine which rupture the end-plate

Compression injuries of the spine may fracture the vertebral end-plate allowing the nucleus pulposus to partially extrude and exposing the proteoglycans in the nucleus pulposus to the intra-osseous blood circulation in the bone marrow of the vertebral body and triggering an auto-immune response. This may induce disc degradation with the end result of disc resorption and narrowing of the intervertebral space, or radial fissures leading to nucleus pulposus herniation (Figure 34).

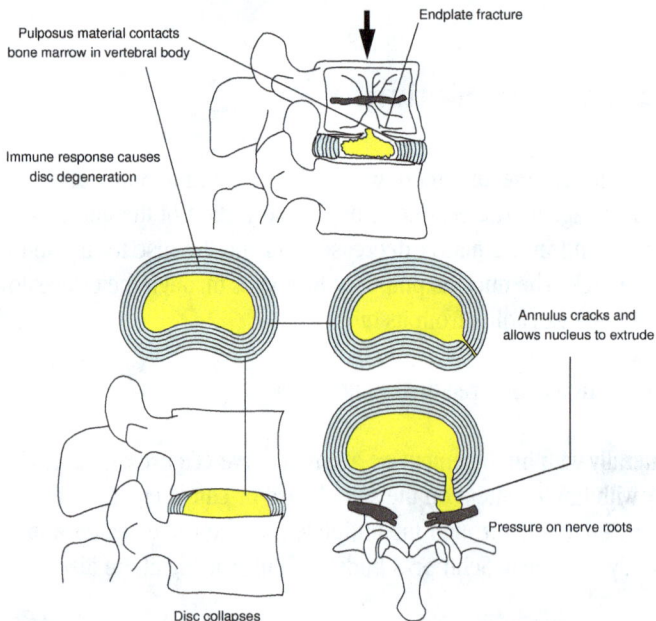

Figure 34. Effects on intervertebral disc of fracture of vertebral end-plate

Anatomical factors influencing spinal nerve compression by intervertebral discs

The spinal cord terminates about the level of L2 vertebra therefore disc prolapse below this level cannot compress the cord, only spinal nerves or the cauda equina.

There are three significant factors:

1. Because the pedicles project from the upper part of the body, the corresponding spinal nerve emerges through its intervertebral foramen above the level of its corresponding disc. Therefore, any impingement of the spinal nerve cannot occur from its own disc but from the disc immediately above. Thus spinal nerve L5 will be compressed by the disc between L4 and 5 vertebrae (Figure 35)
2. The more distal spinal nerves become increasingly vertical in direction. Therefore:
   - L 4 roots can be compressed by disc L3/4
   - L5 roots can be compressed by disc L 4/5 or L5/ S1
   - S1 roots can be compressed by disc L5/S1
3. Central prolapse of disc L 4/5 can compress the cauda equina

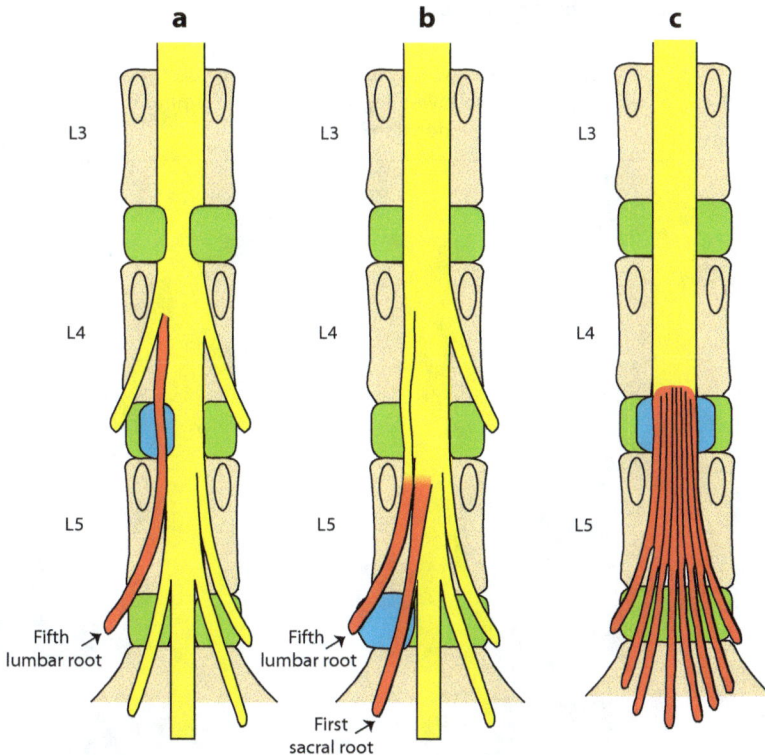

Figure 35. Spinal nerve root compression (red) by disc prolapse (blue) at different levels

PROBLEM No. 3

An Olympic Weight Lifter complains of severe central lower back pain radiating to the left buttock, posterior thigh and down to the mid-lateral leg. The symptoms commenced two days ago whilst doing heavy squats in training. The pain came on suddenly at the bottom (full squat position) of his last lift of a session of 6 sets of 3 repetitions of maximal lifts. He required help from 'spotters' to return the bar to the rack and since then has been unable to bend forward more than a quarter of his normal range of motion due to muscle spasm and pain.

The lifter has a long history of intermittent lower back pain, occasionally radiating to the left buttock, but never this severe.

i)   What is likely to be the primary injury?
ii)   What other structures are implicated?
iii) What is the likely mechanism of injury?
iv)   What other symptoms might be reported and why?

If an MRI scan indicated that the diagnosis was likely to be an L4/5 left lateral disc protrusion, during the clinical examination:

v)   Which spinal nerve is likely to be involved ?
vi)   Which muscles might test as being weak?
vii) Which area/s of skin might have paraesthesia?
viii) Which reflexes might be diminished?

ix)   What might be a possible explanation for the following presentation during the clinical examination; Medial left lower leg paraesthesia, diminution of the patella tendon reflex, weakness of knee extension?

MOVEMENTS OF THE HEAD & SPINE

Head

The most proximal joint in the spine is the articulation between the concave superior articular facets of the atlas and the convex occipital condyles of the skull. These are synovial ellipsoid joints allowing forward flexion and backwards extension of the head, and also slight lateral flexion.

There are three joints between the atlas and axis (the 1st and 2nd cervical vertebrae). On each side there is a plane synovial joint allowing gliding movements between the inferior flat facet of the atlas and the superior flat facet of the axis. In the midline the odontoid process of the axis forms a synovial pivot joint with the anterior arch of the atlas. It is stabilized by the alar (check) ligaments which prevent excessive rotation and by the transverse limb of the cruciate ligament which has a critical role in keeping the odontoid process in contact with the anterior arch (Figure 36a & b). These three joints allow side-to-side rotation movements of the head.

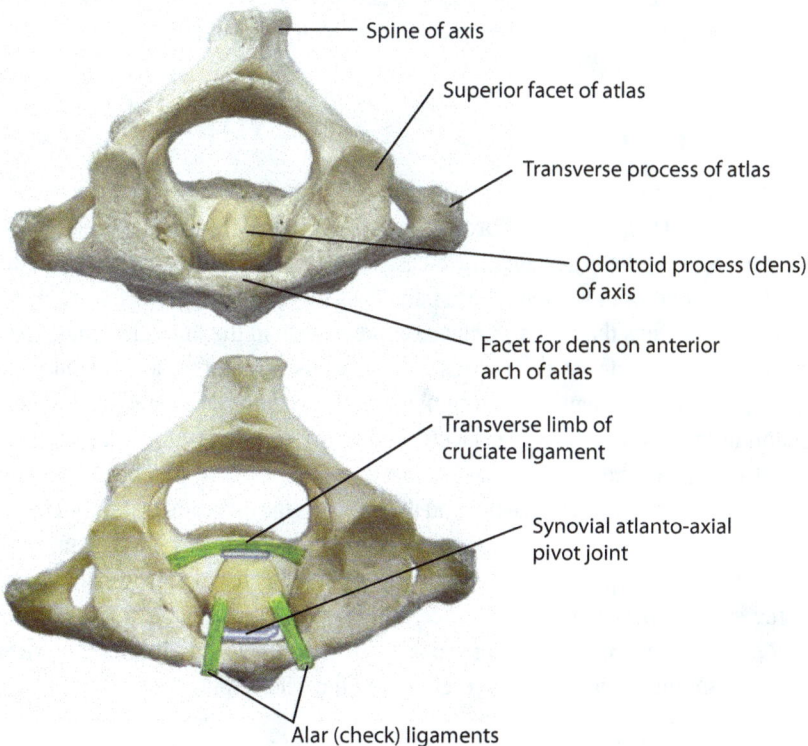

Spine of axis

Superior facet of atlas

Transverse process of atlas

Odontoid process (dens) of axis

Facet for dens on anterior arch of atlas

Transverse limb of cruciate ligament

Synovial atlanto-axial pivot joint

Alar (check) ligaments

Figure 36a. Cruciate ligament and synovial pivot atlanto-axial joint viewed from above

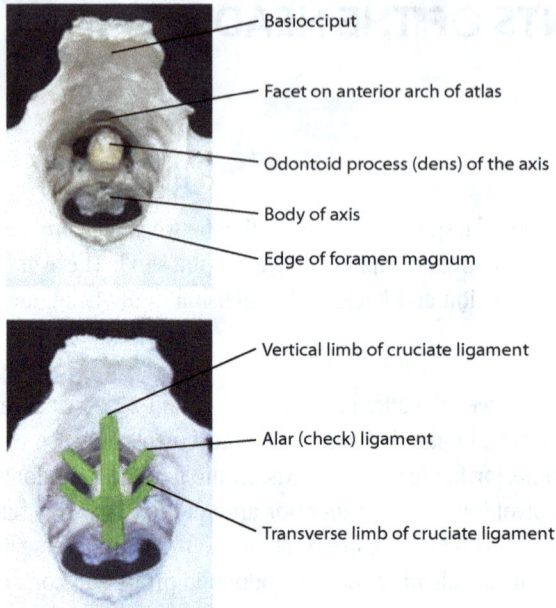

Basiocciput

Facet on anterior arch of atlas

Odontoid process (dens) of the axis

Body of axis

Edge of foramen magnum

Vertical limb of cruciate ligament

Alar (check) ligament

Transverse limb of cruciate ligament

Figure 36b. Cruciate ligament and alar ligaments viewed from posterior cranial fossa looking downwards into spinal canal through foramen magnum

Spine

There are several factors that influence the range and types of movement in the different regions of the spine. Of particular importance is the direction of the facets in the zygapophyseal joints and the shape of the articulating surfaces. The thickness of the intervertebral disc also influences the amount of movement, there being less movement where discs are thin. The presence of ribs restricts the type and range of movements in the thoracic spine. The widest range of movements occurs in the cervical region whilst in the thoracic region rotation is the most significant movement. In the lumbar region rotation is notably restricted due to the direction of the opposing articular facets. The movements and the ranges characterizing the different regions of the spine are summarized in Figure 37. In practice thoraco-lumbar movements are often considered together and this explains the omission of range of movements in the thoracic box in Figure 36. An accurate method of measuring the amount of flexion in the thoraco- lumbar spine is to measure the change in distance between two palpable points using spinous processes as reference points (Harris and Ranson, 2008). Note that between adjacent vertebrae the range of movement is small but it is considerable when these movements are summated in respect of regions and the whole spine.

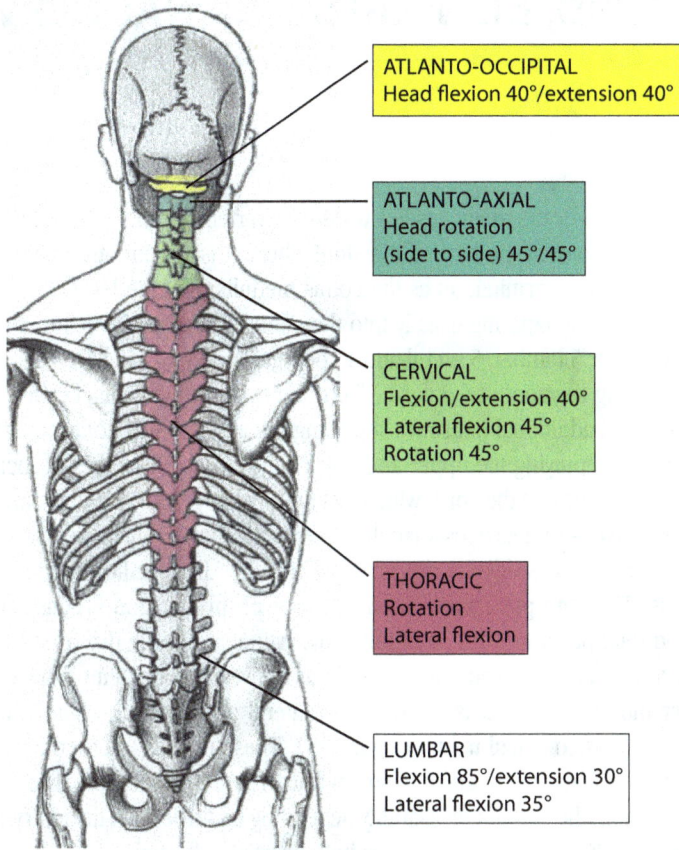

ATLANTO-OCCIPITAL
Head flexion 40°/extension 40°

ATLANTO-AXIAL
Head rotation
(side to side) 45°/45°

CERVICAL
Flexion/extension 40°
Lateral flexion 45°
Rotation 45°

THORACIC
Rotation
Lateral flexion

LUMBAR
Flexion 85°/extension 30°
Lateral flexion 35°

Figure 37. Principal movements at different levels of the spine.
Note: The measurements for range of movements in the lumbar spine also include thoracic
spine contribution

SPINAL CORD, MENINGES & SPINAL NERVES

Spinal Cord:

The spinal cord covered by the meninges lies within the vertebral canal (Figure. 44). It extends from the foramen magnum at the base of the skull where it is continuous with the medulla in the brain-stem down to its termination as the conus medullaris at the level of L2 vertebra. Its overall shape is cylindrical tapering distally into the conus. There are 31 pairs of spinal nerves (8 cervical, 12 thoracic, 5 lumbar, 5 sacral and 1 coccygeal) each of which has roots connecting it to the corresponding segment of the cord. There are two enlargements, cervical and lumbar due to the presence of additional neurones supplying the axons which contribute to the nerves forming the plexuses supplying the upper and lower limbs. The cell bodies of neurones form the grey matter in the centre of the cord which has an 'H' shape, with dorsal, ventral and lateral horns or columns. Axons of neurones form the outer white matter which lie in anterior, lateral and posterior columns. These axons are grouped together in specific 'tracts' which convey specific functions. Thus the posterior columns convey proprioception (conscious sensation of movement and joint position), also light touch, vibration and tactile discrimination, whilst in lateral and anterior columns lie spino-thalamic tracts conveying pain, temperature and general touch. Voluntary motor movement is conveyed in lateral and anterior white columns called lateral and anterior cortico-spinal tracts (Figure 38). These various tracts conveying motor or sensory functions may become disrupted in spinal fractures and dislocation, disc displacements and cord compression, the amount of disability depending on the level of the injury, and whether the anterior or posterior part of the cord, or both parts are affected.

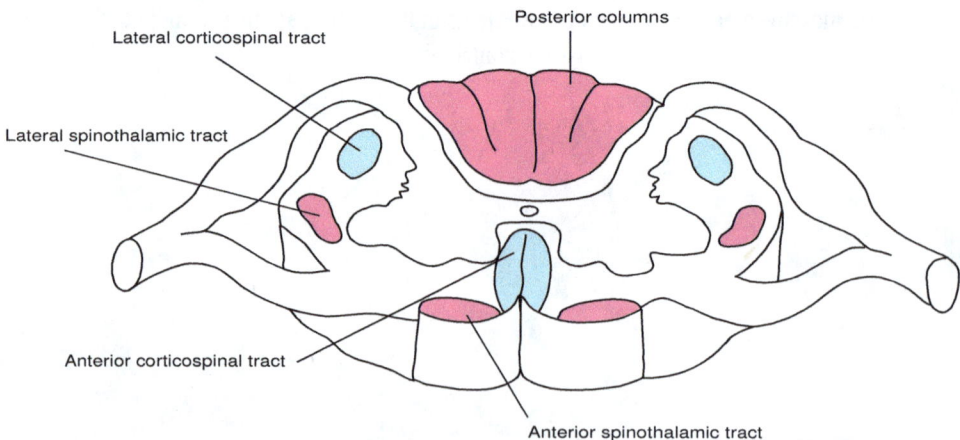

Figure 38. Transverse section of the spinal cord showing principal motor (blue) and sensory (pink) tracts

In the anterior cord syndrome there is damage to tracts in the anterior half of the cord i.e. the cortico-spinal and spino-thalamic tracts causing loss or weakness of voluntary movement and loss of pain and temperature sensation. The posterior columns are unaffected. This syndrome may result from fracture or dislocation of vertebral bodies. In the posterior cord syndrome, there is damage to the tracts in the posterior columns lying in the posterior half of the cord with loss of movement and position sensations, also fine touch and vibration whilst voluntary movements and pain, temperature and course touch are less affected, or unaffected. This syndrome occurs with hyperextension injuries with damage to the neural arch element of the vertebra and herniation of ligamenta flava into the spinal canal.

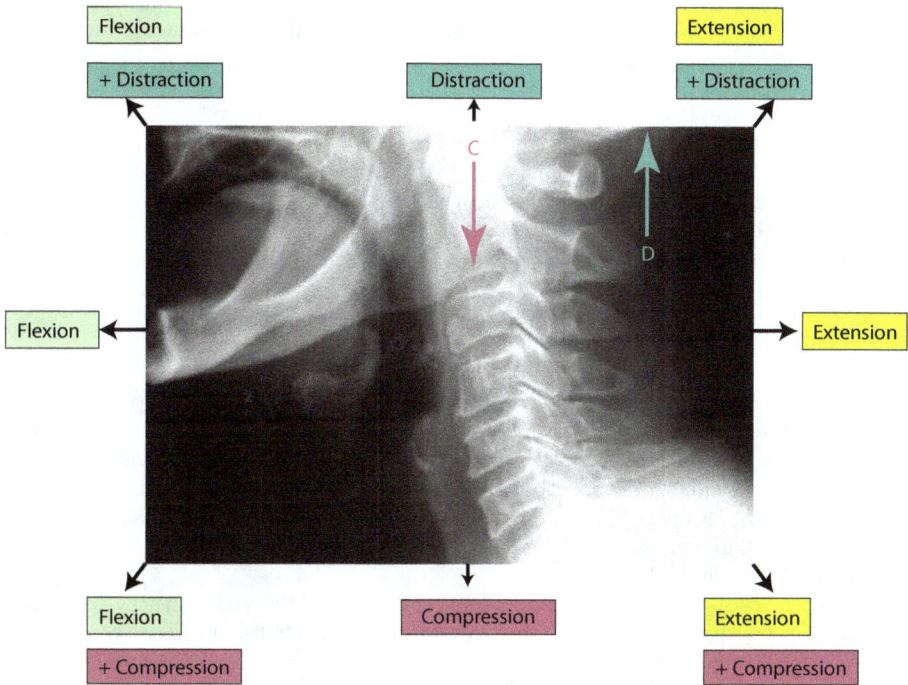

Figure 39. Diagrammatic representation of the different forces acting on the upper cervical spine which influence the type of fracture produced in the Atlas or Axis vertebra

The cord is particularly susceptible to damage to the atlas or axis vertebrae involving compression or stretching (distraction) with concomitant ischaemia. An additional factor is whether flexion or extension accompany these distortions (Figure 39) since this will also determine the type of vertebral damage. In severe compression, burst fractures of the vertebral body may occur. If there is an element of torsion this may result in subluxation or dislocation of facet joints (Figure 42). Types of injury to the atlas and axis are shown in Figures 40 and 41. Of particular note are dislocation of the atlas from the occipital condyles, fractures of both arches of the atlas, fractures of the dens, body and pedicles of the axis with displacement due to rupture of the cruciate ligament which retains the dens against the anterior arch of the atlas.

The range of injuries is comprehensively illustrated in cranio-cervical trauma with injuries around C1-C2 complex by Frymoyer *et al.*, (1997). C1-2 compression related fractures can occur in tackling- sports such as rugby or American football when the crown of the tackler's head is driven into an opponent. A further example of compression injury may occur in equestrian sports when a rider lands on the crown of the head after falling from a horse.

Problem No. 4

A 34 year old Australian Rules football player's cervical spine is forcefully extended and side-flexed to the left when he makes the tackle on an opponent running towards him. His neck is again forcefully extended when he lands onto his back completing the tackle. He immediately complains to the on-field medical attendant that he has severe left lower cervical pain radiating to the region of the left upper trapezius.

i.   What structures might be the source of the left lower cervical pain?
ii. The footballer also complains of some numbness, pain, pins and needles and weakness affecting his entire right upper limb. What might be the mechanism for these symptoms?
iii. During the on-field assessment how could weakness of the muscles associated with the following nerve roots be assessed?
iv. During the on-field assessment where would the dermatome associated with the following nerve roots be assessed?
   C7
   C6
   C8
v.   Although there is some residual left neck pain the player has full cervical range of motion and the right sided symptoms resolve within 2 minutes and the medical attendant clears the player to return to play. The next day he continues to complain of left lower cervical pain with active cervical extension, left side-flexion and left rotation. There is tenderness over the left C6/7 articular pillar. X-ray shows no bony injury and there are no neurological signs or symptoms?
   i. What is the likely clinical diagnosis
vi. The player also complains of deep soreness at the front of the neck with active cervical flexion and passive cervical extension. What structures might be injured and why?

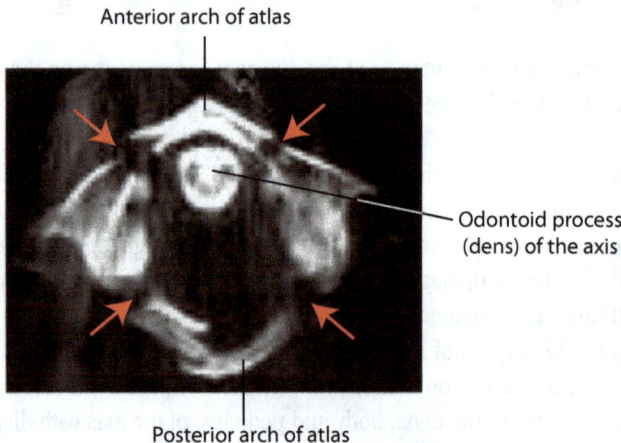

Anterior arch of atlas

Odontoid process (dens) of the axis

Posterior arch of atlas

Figure 40. CT scan showing fractures (red arrows) of both arches of the Atlas (Jefferson fracture)

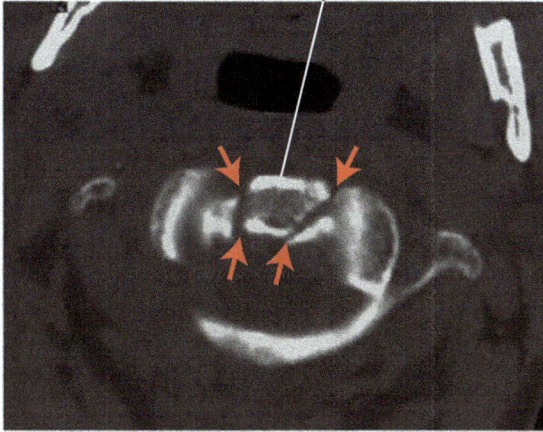

Odontoid process (dens) of the axis

Figure 41. CT scan of fractures (red arrows) of the dens of the Axis (Figures 39 and 40 by kind permission of Michael Rissing ,Senior student, Dept. of Radiology, University of South Carolina Medical School)

Problem No. 5

A 26 year old female equestrian rider is thrown from her bucking horse during a schooling session. The top of her helmeted head hits the ground with her inverted body almost vertical. The rider does not lose consciousness and sits up on the ground where she is found holding onto her helmet with both hands. She refuses to let go fearing 'her head feels like it will fall off' until paramedics arrive and extricate her into an ambulance using a spinal board and rigid collar.

i.   Following X-radiography investigation at the hospital doctors explain that the woman has a 'Jefferson Fracture'. Which bones are involved? Describe the X-radiograph appearance of this type of fracture?
ii. What other investigation is likely to be conducted following the X-radiograph findings and for what purpose?
iii. Why would the rider have been apprehensive about letting go of her grip on her own head?
iv. Describe the mechanism by which this type of injury could occur in another sport?
v.   Nine months after surgical fixation of the fracture the woman returns to riding yet is troubled by severe occipital headaches that come on after more than 10 mins in the saddle. Which structures that may have been injured during the initial injury might be a source of the head pain?

Injuries in these upper cervical vertebrae are also seen in diving accidents and in gymnasts. About 50% of cervical spine injuries involve the lower vertebrae, C6 and C7.

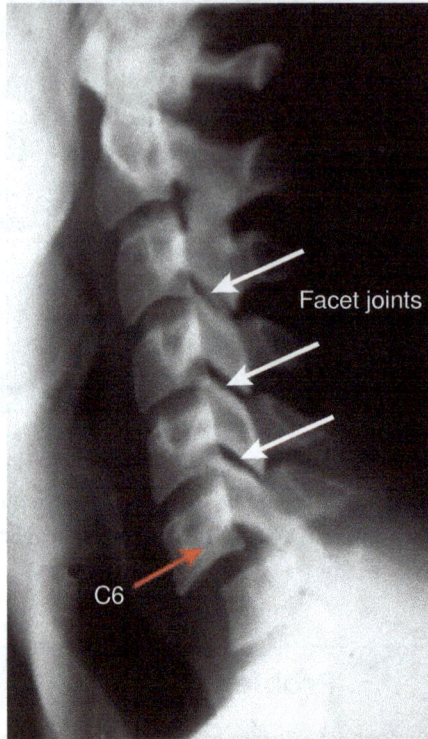

Figure 42. X-Radiograph of fracture/dislocation of C6 vertebra (red arrow)

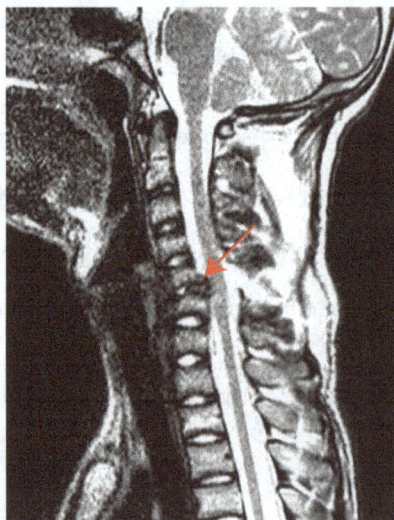

Figure 43. Sagittal MRI scan of neck showing ventral cord compression due to traumatic retro-pulsion of the C4/5 disc (arrow) following forced neck flexion during a rugby scrum

Problem No. 6

The collapse of a scrum causes a Rugby forward's neck to be forced into full flexion under the weight of several players pushing in front of, and behind him. The team doctor attends him on the field and finds the player lying on his back unable to move.

i.   What would be the doctor's primary first aid concerns?
ii.   What manoeuvre should a first aid provider perform in this type of scenario?
iii.   How should the player be evacuated from the field?
iv.   Given the mechanism of injury, which specific tissues might have been injured (list a minimum of four)?
v.   What spinal level is most likely affected if further off-field assessment reveals that the player; is able to diaphragmatically breathe, can feel painful stimuli over lateral arm but has complete loss of sensation from the elbow down and from the chest down, has full power of shoulder abduction but mild weakness of elbow flexion, is unable to extend the elbow and has no voluntary movement in the hand, trunk or lower limbs?
vi.   What would be the most appropriate radiological investigation to rule out or delineate the extent of any cervical fracture?

Effects of damage at different levels in the spinal cord

Severe damage in the upper cervical cord (C1-3) produces total paralysis of all 4 limbs, and loss of all sensation below the level of the damage. Also, paralysis of respiratory movements by the diaphragm, requires ventilation of the patient. In mid- cervical (C5) damage (Figures 42 and 43) diaphragm movement is present but there is weakness or paralysis and wasting of the shoulder muscles and in the proximal arm, together with loss of reflexes in the upper limbs. Hand function is lost. There is complete paralysis of the lower limbs and complete sensory loss below the level of the damage.

In upper thoracic cord damage (below T1) the upper limbs are little affected but there is total paraplegia involving both lower limbs and complete sensory loss in the trunk and lower limbs below the level of the damage. At levels T1- 12 there is lack of control of abdominal wall muscles, being more marked with damage at the higher levels.

In lumbar cord damage there is weakness and muscle wasting in the lower limbs with loss of reflexes together with sensory loss in the limbs and trunk below the level of the lesion. Damage to the most distal part of the cord, the conus medullaris, produces 'saddle-shaped' anaesthesia in the region of the buttocks and perineum together with loss of control of bladder and rectal sphincters. In the male there may be erectile dysfunction.

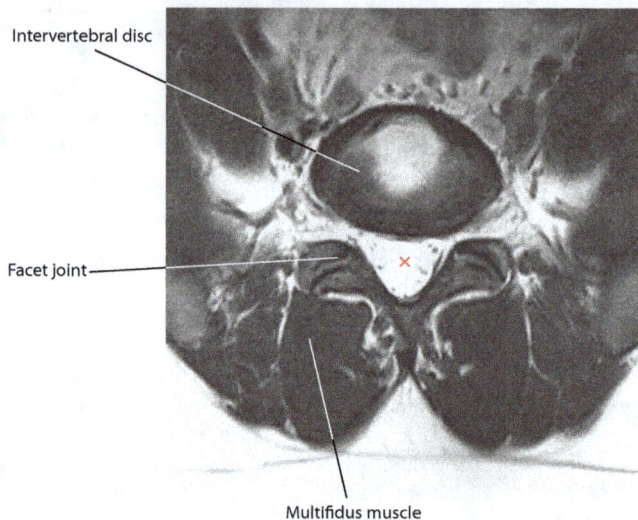

Figure 44. Cauda equina & meninges (red cross) with related structures

Thoraco-lumbar flexion distraction injuries

This type of injury occurs in athletes who land forcefully on their feet with concurrent sudden acute forced forward flexion of the trunk. The thoraco-lumbar spine is particularly vulnerable. It is seen in athletes and also in seat lap-belt injuries. There is acute disc disruption and protrusion which may be so severe that there is cord compression with development of paraplegia and girdle anaesthesia. An MRI scan illustrating this type of injury is shown in Figure 45.

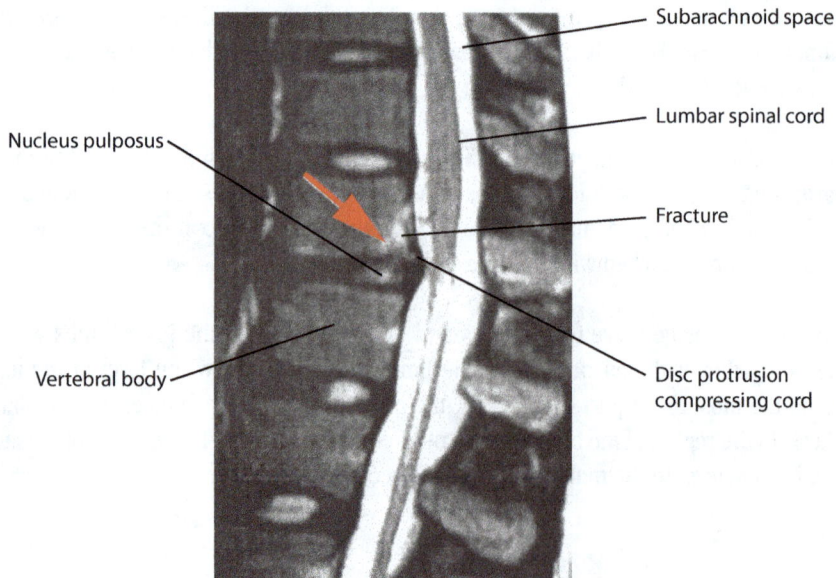

Figure 45. MRI scan showing distal spinal cord compression by a disc protrusion and an infero-posterior vertebral body fracture (red arrow)

Problem No. 7

A 60 year old female parachutist suffers severe mid-thoracic pain following a very heavy miss-timed landing onto her feet. Her pain is reproduced with trunk flexion, deep breathing, coughing and sneezing.

i.   What type of fracture pattern might be associated with this mechanism
ii. Why might this particular sports person be susceptible to fracture
iii. What other mid thoracic structures might have been injured due to this mechanism

Meninges

The meninges surround the spinal cord as three layers. The innermost, the pia mater, is thin and vascular and intimately covers the cord. External to this is the arachnoid mater separated from the pia by the subarachnoid space containing cerebrospinal fluid (CSF). This space extends beyond the termination of the cord to reach the sacral canal where it terminates at the level of S2. This extension is called the lumbar sac and contains the cauda equina which comprises the lumbar, sacral and coccygeal nerve roots. The arachnoid mater is adjacent to the outermost layer of the meninges, the dura mater which is thick and strong. As the dorsal and ventral roots of the spinal nerves pass laterally to reach the corresponding intervertebral foramen they evaginate the dura and arachnoid layers pulling them outwards like a sleeve, the dura mater being continuous with the epineurium of the spinal nerve. The evagination also includes the subarachnoid space containing the CSF which bathes the nerve roots and the dorsal root ganglion (Figure 47). If nerve roots are torn by traction injuries on limb plexuses the meningeal sheaths may also be torn causing CSF to leak outside the spinal canal and track along tissue planes some distance from the spine. Also dural adhesions in the intervertebral foramen or adjacent paravertebral muscles may cause pain along the distribution of the spinal nerve particularly when it is stretched.

Spinal Nerves

Each of the 31 pairs of spinal nerves has two roots, dorsal and ventral, attached to the spinal cord. The dorsal root contains sensory fibres (pain, temperature, touch, pressure and proprioception). As the dorsal root passes laterally to reach the intervertebral foramen a small swelling (ganglion) marks the location of the cell bodies of the sensory neurones whose central processes comprise the dorsal root. The ventral root contains motor axons passing to voluntary muscles. From the T1 to the L2 segments the ventral root also contains sympathetic fibres which supply blood vessels, sweat glands and small erector pilae muscles of hairs. In the intervertebral foramen the nerve roots and dorsal root ganglion lie in an evagination of the

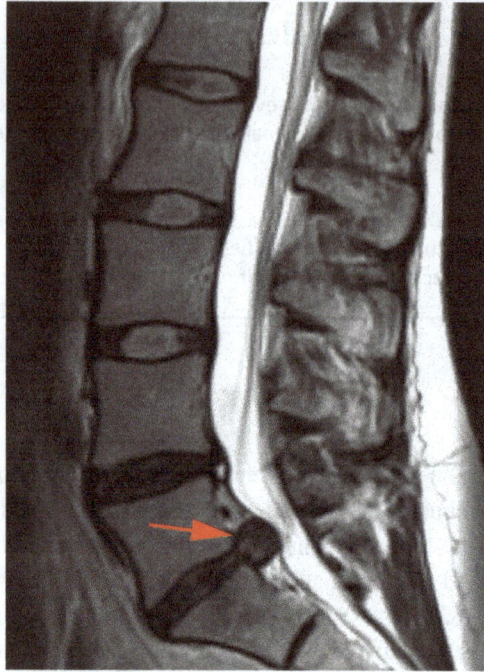

Figure 46a. Sagittal MRI scan showing disc protrusion at level L5/S1 compressing the cauda equina (red arrow)

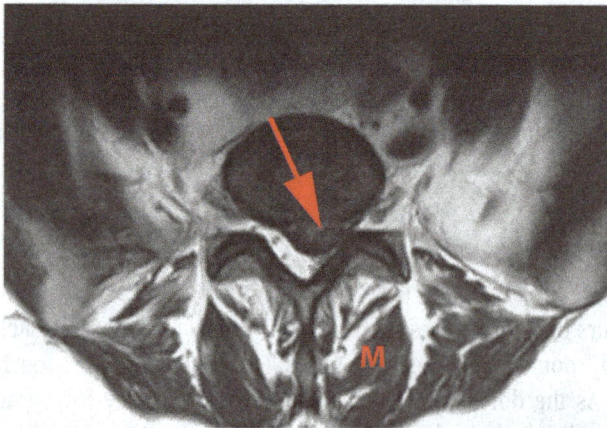

Figure 46b. Axial MRI scan showing postero-lateral disc protrusion at L5/S1 (red arrow) also atrophy with fat and fibrous tissue (white material) infiltration of the adjacent multifidus muscle (M)

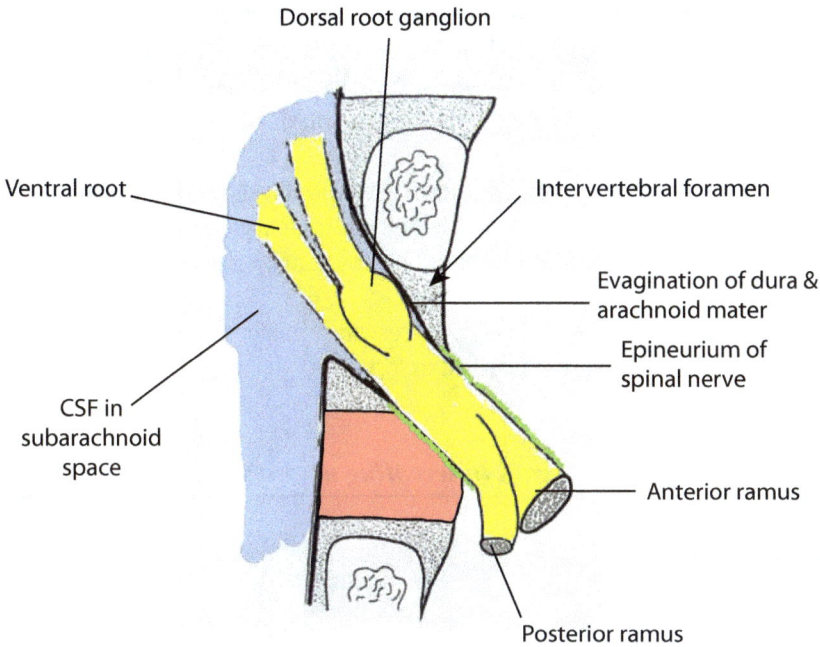

Figure 47. Dural sheath evagination in intervertebral foramen

outer meninges where they are bathed in CSF before finally emerging from the intervertebral foramen as the spinal nerve at which point the dural sheath merges with the epineurium covering the spinal nerve.

Nerve roots or the spinal nerve may be compressed by prolapsed discs or articular facet encroachment in the intervertebral foramen resulting in sensory (pain, tingling and numbness) and motor (weakness or paralysis) changes.

Segmental innervation of muscles, myotomes and spinal reflexes

When examining for the level of suspected nerve root compression or cord damage, specific limb muscles can be tested (Table 1) or groups of muscles (myotomes) controlling joint movements may be tested (Table 2).

Concerning myotomes, there is a logical progression down the spinal cord of the segments and roots involved in the movements of the joints from the proximal to the distal part of the limb.

In the case of the lower limb there is an orderly progression down the limb, one movement being controlled from two segments and the opposite movement by the next two segments. As the limb is examined progressively, distally each set of movements changes by one segment e.g. hip flexion/extension L2,3/L4,5 but knee extension/flexion L3,4/L5, S1.

Concerning the upper limb myotomes, the arrangement for the more proximal joints is similar to that in the lower limb but for the more distal joints movements in one direction, and also the opposite, are controlled from the same segments e.g. finger flexion/extension C7,8.

At certain levels, due to disruption of either the sensory or motor component of the reflex arc, spinal reflexes (Table 3) may be diminished or lost.

Table 1. Segments of spinal cord innervating muscles

Upper limb

Deltoid	C5
Biceps	C5/6
Serratus anterior	C5/6/7
Abductor pollicis longus	C6/7
Triceps	C6/7/8
Extensor pollicis longus & Extensor digitorum	C7
Flexor carpi ulnaris & Flexor pollicis longus	C8/T1
Adductor pollicis	T1

Lower limb

Psoas major	L1/2
Adductor longus	L2/3
Quadriceps femoris	L3/4
Tibialis anterior	L4/5
Peroneii	L4/5
Extensor hallucis longus	L5
Extensor digitorum longus	L5/S1
Calf	S1
Hamstrings	L5, S1/2
Glutei	S1/2
Anal & urinary sphincters	S3/4

Table 2. Myotomes

Upper limb

Shoulder	- Abduction + lateral rotation	C5
	- Adduction + medial rotation	C6/7
Elbow	- Flexion	C5/6
	- Extension	C7/8
	- Supination/pronation	C6
Wrist	- Flexion/extension	C6/7
Fingers	- Flexion/extension	C7/8
Hand short muscles		T1

Lower limb

Hip	- Flexion+adduction+medial rotation	L2/3
	- Extension+abduction+lateral rotation	L4/5
Knee	- Extension	L3/4
	- Flexion	L5, S1
Ankle	- Dorsiflexion (extension)	L4/5
	- Plantarflexion	S1/2
Foot	- Inversion	L4
	- Eversion	L5, S1

Table 3. Spinal reflexes

Trunk

Epigastric	T7
Umbilical	T10
Cremaster	L1

Upper limb

Biceps	C5/6
Triceps	C7/8
Brachioradialis/supinator	C6

Lower limb

Knee (patellar tendon)	L3/4
Adductor Longus	L3/4
Hamstring (deep tendon)	L5/S1
Ankle (Achilles tendon)	S1/2

Cauda equina compression

Since the cauda equina contains spinal nerve roots from the level of L2 down to S5 and Coccygeal 1, pressure on the cauda (Figures 46a and b) can result in sensory impairment, muscle weakness and diminished reflexes, the extent depending on which roots are compressed. Clinically the patient may present with neurogenic claudication, motor and sensory symptoms characteristically worsening with exercise but often relieved by activities involving lumbar flexion such as uphill walking. Since spinal nerves S2, 3 and 4 contain parasympathetic fibres (nervi erigentes) an additional feature of pressure on these nerves may be disturbances of bladder and anal sphincter control and possibly erectile disturbances.

Important local branches: Two nerves are specially important. These are:

- As it passes posteriorly, the dorsal ramus of the spinal nerve lies very close to the synovial facet joint and supplies it with sensory fibres (Figure 48).

- The sinuvertebral nerve arises from the ventral ramus but is recurrent, entering the intervertebral foramen to supply the dural sleeve, the outer layers of the intervertebral disc, and the anterior and posterior longitudinal ligaments (Figure 48). Note, although arising from the ventral ramus it is sensory in function, containing pain and proprioceptive fibres, also grey rami vasomotor sympathetic fibres.

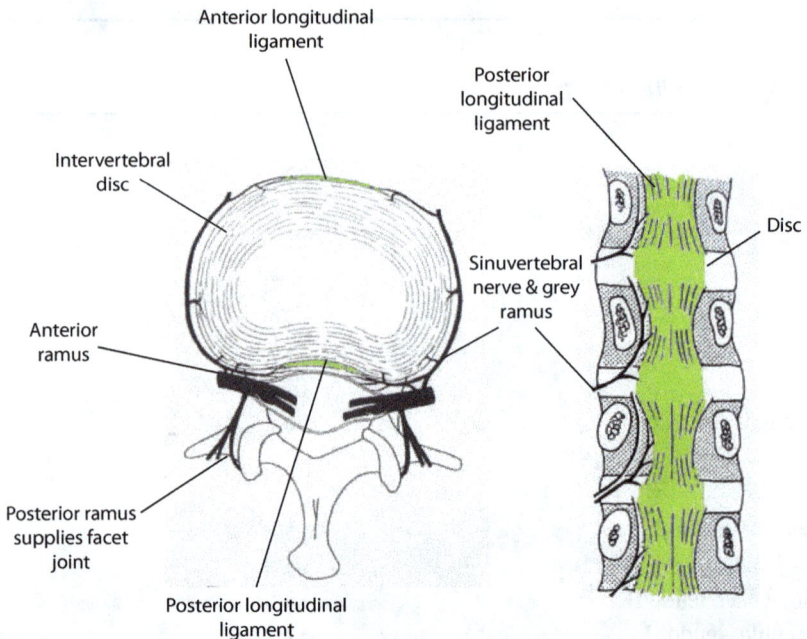

Figure 48. The nerve supply to an intervertebral disc and longitudinal ligaments. Reproduced with permission from Clinical anatomy of the lumbar spine, Fig. 9.9 by N.Bogduk and LT Twomey, Churchill Livingstone , Copyright Elsevier 1987

The normal annulus fibrosus cells are a source of neurotrophins (NT), including neural growth factor (NGF) and contain NT receptors. In degenerating discs, often associated with pain, the NT levels are much increased and there is also a *big increase in nerve fibres* in the disc, the result of in-growth from existing nerves in response to increased levels of NGF. It is also thought that NGF may act directly on pain fibres and neurones to trigger hyperalgesic responses (Garcia-Cosamalon *et al.*2010).

Dermatomes

From sensory endings in the skin nerve fibres pass centrally via anterior and posterior rami of spinal nerves. The anterior rami supply the upper and lower limbs and the ventral part of the trunk whilst the posterior rami supply the dorsal part of the trunk. On entering the spinal canal through the intervertebral foramen sensory fibres pass from the spinal nerve into its dorsal root ganglion . From the ganglion sensory fibres continue centrally through the dorsal root to enter the spinal cord.

A dermatome is the area of skin that is supplied by sensory nerve fibres from the anterior or posterior ramus of **a single** spinal nerve. The dermatomes are arranged in a regular sequence as segments on the trunk (Figure 48) and also in the limbs. Usually their territories overlap e.g. T10 dermatome overlaps with T9 and T11, so that individual dermatomes are not precise. However in the limbs there is greater precision because as the foetal limb bud grows, some segments move to the distal part of the limb. Consequently non-adjacent segments meet at the surface along lines designated as axial lines (Figure 49).

When examining for dermatome deficiency certain features should be noted in the various regions. On examining the ventral part of the trunk note that the C4 dermatome meets the T2 dermatome at the level of the sterno-manubrial angle along the line of the 2nd rib. The 'missing' dermatomes are located in the upper limb being supplied by branches of the brachial plexus. The dermatome at the costal margin is T7, at the umbilicus it is T10 and in the supra-pubic region L1. There are therefore a total of seven dermatomes between the costal margin and the pubis, three above the umbilicus and three below. When examining the trunk posteriorly dermatomes are supplied by posterior rami and extend as far as the angles of the ribs except for the shoulder region where C4 and T2 dermatomes reach as far laterally as the acromion process of the scapula.

Concerning limb dermatomes, in the upper limb there is an orderly progression from C5 to T1 (recall the roots of the brachial plexus) passing down the pre-axial border of the limb to the hand where T7 (the middle root of the plexus) is located and then back up the postaxial border to the axilla and the T2 dermatome. In the lower limb the dermatomes are traced distally down the anterior aspect of the limb to the foot and then proximally up the posterior aspect of the limb to the gluteal region. The L1 dermatome lies just below the crease of the groin over the femoral triangle, L2 lies mid thigh and L3 lies in the lower thigh above the patella. The S1 dermatome corresponds to the footprint and is the area on which a person stands, the S2 dermatome passes extensively from the heel up the back of the leg and thigh to the gluteal region, the S3 & 4 dermatomes are in the gluteal region and correspond to the area upon which a person sits, whilst S5 is in the peri-anal region.

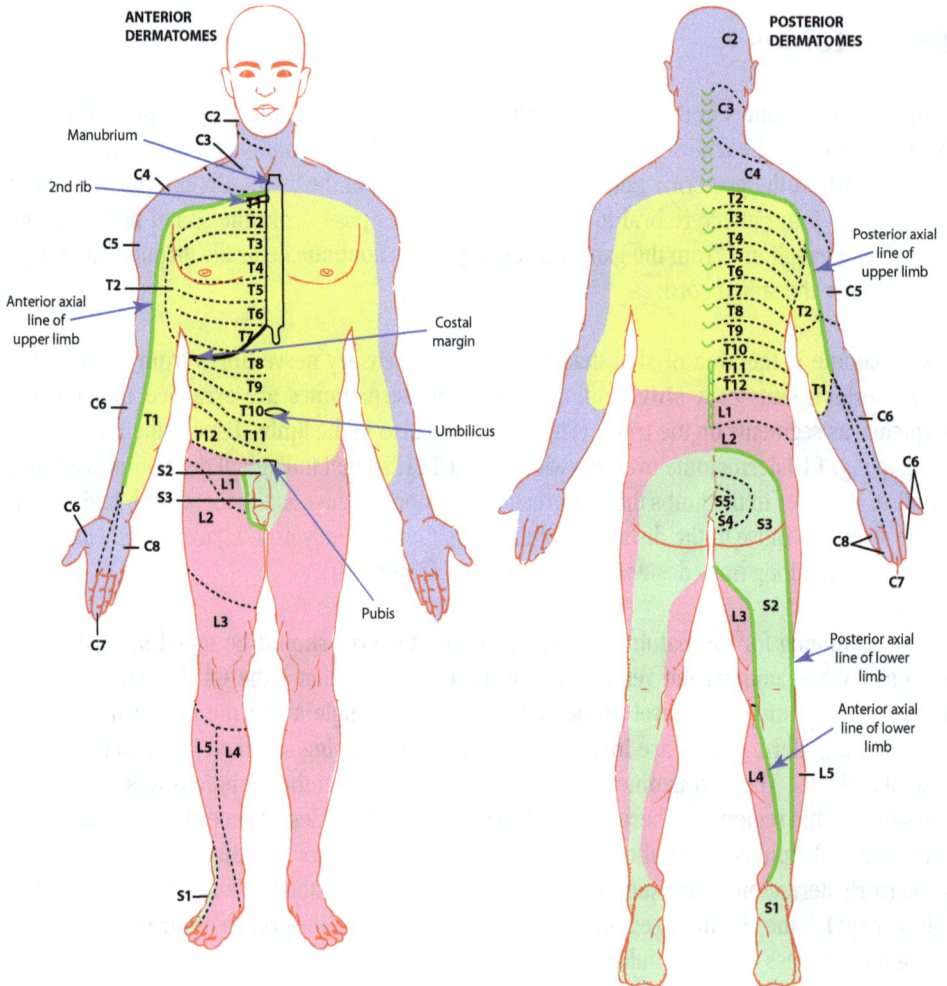

Figure 49. Dermatomes of the trunk and limbs

Problem No. 8

A doctor at a car race is asked to evaluate a 30 year old male driver who has recently changed from Indy Car racing on banked oval circuits with left hand turns only, to touring car racing on circuits characterised by numerous left and right sharp bends. During practice and races he is experiencing left sided neck and arm pain.

i.   What influence might the type of track play in this presentation?
ii. The driver presents with a painful limitation of right cervical rotation of 25° and side flexion of 10°. What ROM of cervical rotation and side flexion would normally be expected?
iii. What might be causing the limitation of rotation?
iv. What risk factors would a race car driver have for cervical injury?
v.   What might be the cause of examination findings of; right sided diminished biceps and brachioradialis reflexes, mild weakness of right elbow flexion and numbness over the radial forearm and hand?
vi. What are the possible sites and causes of cervical nerve root compression?
vii. Which nerve of the brachial plexus is likely to be under most tension due to a driving position of right cervical rotation and side-flexion, left shoulder abduction, elbow extension and wrist flexion whilst changing gears in a right hand drive car during a right hand turn?

Muscles

Muscles of the back are arranged into two groups, superficial and deep.

The superficial muscles are extrinsic and it is more relevant to consider them in detail in studies of the shoulder, upper limb, and neck. They anchor the shoulder girdle and proximal part of the upper limb to the dorsum of the trunk. They include trapezius, levator scapulae and the rhomboids attaching to the scapula or clavicle and latissimus dorsi to the upper end of the humerus (Figure 50). They are all supplied by anterior rami of spinal nerves. Those attaching to the shoulder girdle may be involved in the cervical postural and muscle shortening syndromes.

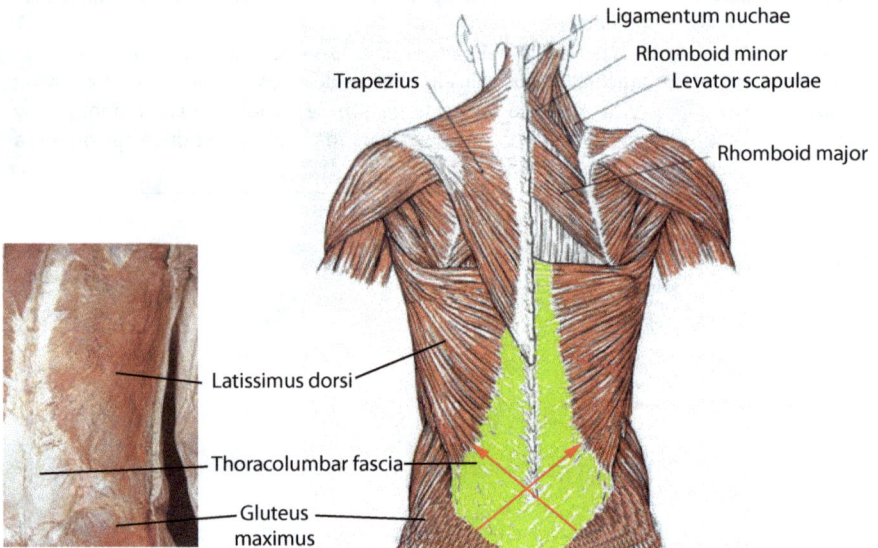

Figure 50. The thoraco-lumbar fascia linking the gluteus maximus to the superficial back muscles (arrows)

The deep muscles are described as intrinsic and collectively as the erector spinae group (Figure 51). They are antigravity muscles that keep the spine and head upright, being particularly large and powerful in the lumbo-sacral region and neck. They occupy the gutter between the spinous processes of the vertebrae and the posterior angles of the ribs (Figures 51 and 52). Their nerve supply is from the posterior rami of spinal nerves. They are arranged into two groups, superficial and deep. The superficial are longitudinal and form three columns as they sweep superiorly (Figure 51) but have a common origin inferiorly, the sacro-spinalis covered by the thick thoraco-lumbar fascia (Figure 50). This fascia continues laterally into the flank giving attachment to the transversus abdominis and internal oblique muscles of the abdominal wall. Therefore, contraction of these muscles as when lifting may significantly pull on the fascia and thereby increase tension in the erector spinae group supporting the spine.

The superficial group extend over considerable lengths of the spine and cross numerous vertebrae. The deep group occupy the gutter between the spinous processes and the transverse processes (Figures 52a & b) but extend over shorter lengths and span fewer vertebrae, the deepest only extending between adjacent vertebrae. They are oblique in direction.

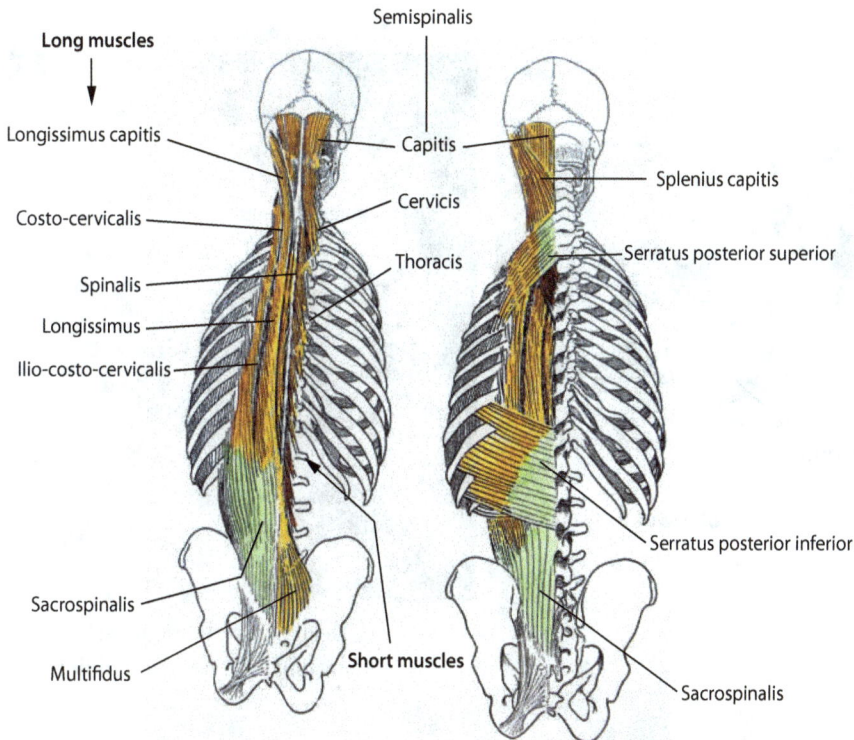

Figure 51. Deep back muscles

Coordinated contraction of the superficial longitudinal muscles on both sides produces extension of the spine. Acting unilaterally they produce lateral flexion. The shorter deeper group are essentially postural in function helping to stabilise local segments of the spine but also produce local rotation, except for in the lumbar region. That these deeper muscles may have an important and special role as feed-back sensors, monitoring and controlling spinal movement and stability, is emphasized by their *high content of muscle spindles* (Nitz and Peck 1986, Buxton and Peck, 1989). Thus, anything affecting the integrity of these muscles such as surgery, or pain inhibition (Hides *et al.*, 2011) has obvious implications for spinal stability with possible repercussions for sporting performance and injury risk.

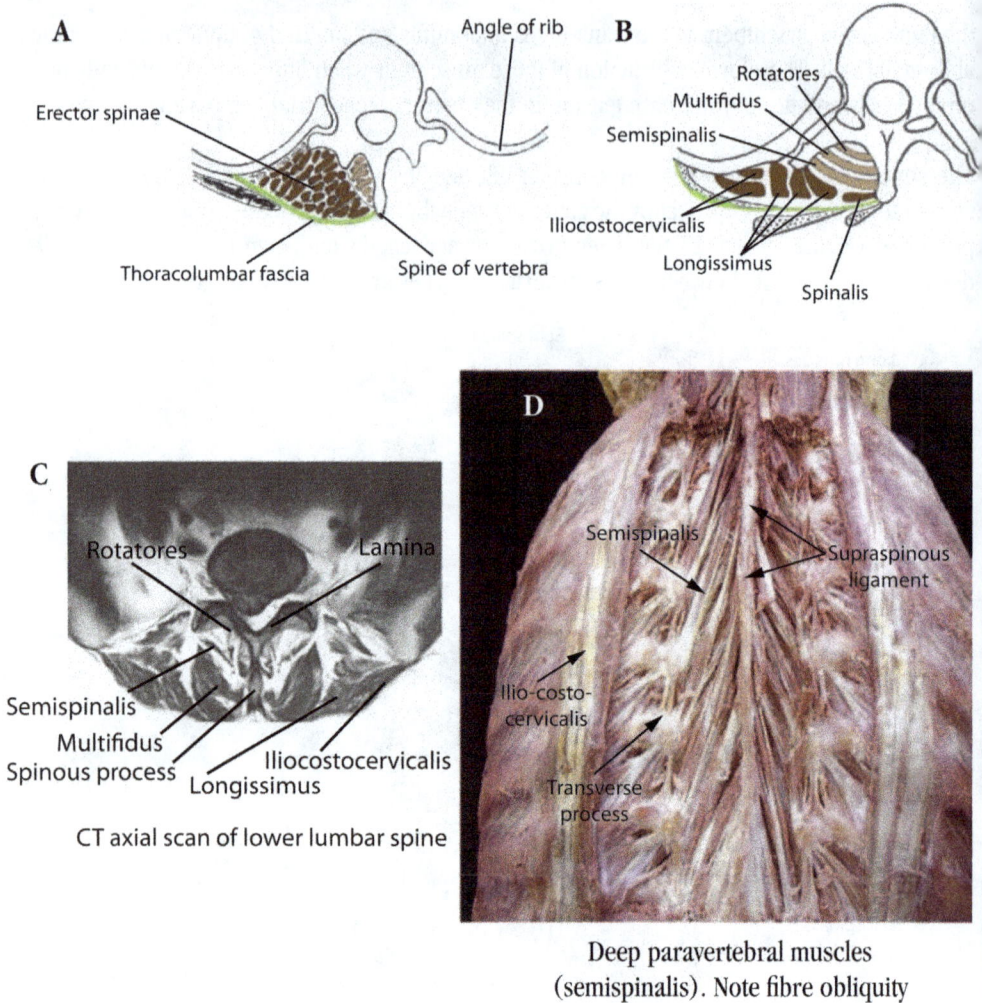

Deep paravertebral muscles
(semispinalis). Note fibre obliquity

Figure 52. Location of deep muscles of the back

The mechanisms of spinal control (Reeves *et al*., 2011) along with methods for training and rehabilitating the spine to minimize injury risk remain controversial. Popular concepts focusing on exercise aimed at 'normalising' the timing of isolated low intensity activation of specific deep muscles such as the transversus abdominis and multifidi, have recently been challenged (Lederman, 2011). However, comprehensive evidence-based exercise rehabilitation guidelines for sports related back pain and injury are not yet available.

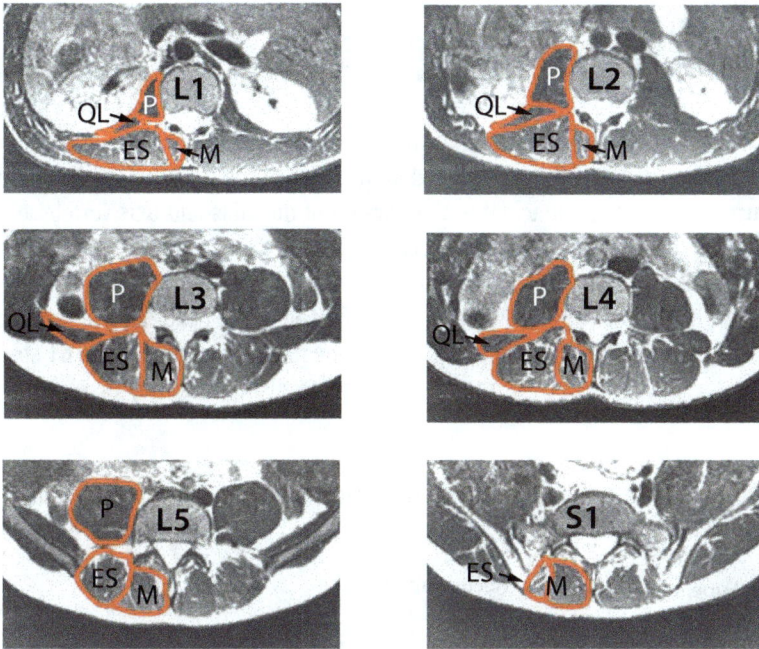

Figure 53. Axial MRI scans showing the lumbar paraspinal muscles at L1 to S1 vertebral levels. Psoas major (P), Quadratus Lumborum (QL), Erector Spinae -combined Iliocostalis and Longissimus (ES) and Multifidus (M)

Problem No. 9

A 28 year old female field hockey player presents with localised left sided pain in the region of the thoraco-lumbar junction first felt on waking the day after a match played the previous evening. She cannot recall feeling any pain during or immediately after the match. However, an opponent did push her in the back with her stick in the second half. The deep achy pain that becomes sharp with certain movements is localised to an area of approximately 3cm in diameter centered 5cm lateral to the T10 spinous process.

i.   If the athlete has discomfort and weakness with active trunk extension in the prone position what muscle group might be implicated?
ii. If the athlete has discomfort and weakness with active trunk side flexion to the left when lying on her right side what muscles might be implicated?
iii. Which joints lying deep to the region of symptoms might be involved if the athlete has painful restriction of left trunk rotation and left trunk side-flexion?
iv. What pathology might be suspected if the athlete's pain is reproduced with coughing and sneezing?
v.   What examination technique might be used to test for lower rib fracture?
vi. Why might it be prudent to examine a urine specimen in this case?

Suboccipital muscles

The splenius capitis and semispinalis capitis, covered by the upper fibres of trapezius, form the bulk of the palpable muscle mass at the back of the neck and overlie the suboccipital muscles which are short and deeply placed at the back of the neck below the occiput of the skull (Figure 54). They are attached to the dorsum of the atlas and axis vertebrae, spanning the gap between these vertebrae and the occiput. They are in pairs, two are oblique (inferior and superior), and two are straight (rectus capitis minor and major). Acting at the atlanto-occipital joint they produce extension and lateral flexion of the head, and at the atlanto-axial joints they produce rotation. They are supplied by the posterior ramus of the C1 spinal nerve. Fractures of the posterior arch of the atlas and spine of the axis may disrupt the occipital muscles.

Splenius capitis, acting bilaterally, extends the head. Acting on one side it laterally flexes and rotates the head to the same side. Semispinalis capitis, acting together, extend the head.

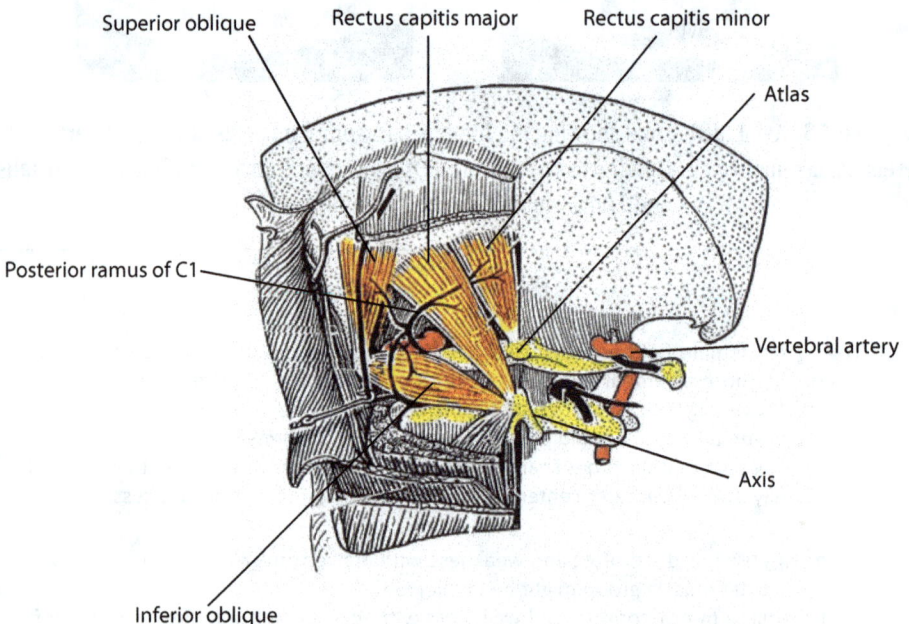

Figure 54. The suboccipital region and suboccipital muscles

Other muscles producing movements of the head and spine

These muscles are summarized below but with the exception of the prevertebral muscles are not intrinsic to the spine and should be studied in detail in relation to their regional anatomy.

The prevertebral group are mostly postural in function and are minor in comparison with the much larger group of antigravity extensors of the neck.

Trapezius (upper fibres)	Extension of head
Sternocleidomastoid:	Flexion of head
	Lateral flexion of head
	Rotation of head to the opposite side
Scalenes:	Lateral flexion of the cervical spine
	Forward flexion and contralateral rotation
	(scalenus anterior only)
Longus capitis & cervicis	Forward flexion of cervical spine
(prevertebral muscles)	Lateral flexion (unilateral action)
Psoas major	Flexion of lumbar spine (bilateral)
	Lateral flexion (unilateral)
Quadratus lumborum:	Lateral flexion of lumbar spine
Rectus abdominis:	Flexion of thoracic & lumbar spine (bilateral)
	Lateral flexion of thoracic and lumbar spine (unilateral)

Abdominal flank muscles- internal oblique + external oblique on contralateral side acting in functional continuity through rectus sheath: Rotate thoracic spine

Myo-fascial continuity between the back and adjacent regions

A recent concept that proposes a system of myo-fascial continuity between regions is termed 'anatomy trains' (Myers, 2008). For example, within this concept the 'superficial back line' (Figure 55) is said to be able to be traced contiguously from the lower limb through the back to the head. It is proposed that this 'train' could convey forces produced in the powerful lower limb muscles such as those of the calf and posterior thigh to the erector spinae via the sacro-tuberous ligament and sacral fascia. The implication for injury prevention and treatment may be that dysfunction in one region e.g. the posterior lower limb, may be linked to pain or injury in another, such as the back.

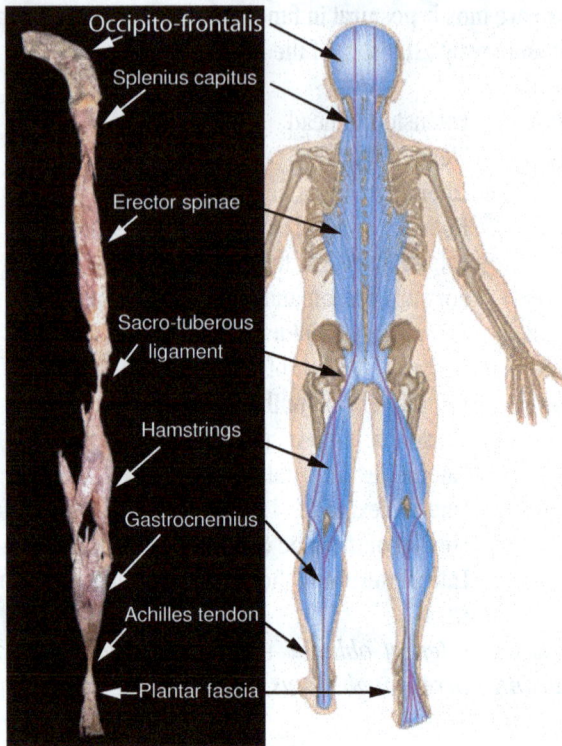

Figure 55. The 'superficial back line' anatomy train

References

Buxton DF and Peck D (1989) Neuromuscular spindles relative to joint complexities *Clin. Anat.* **2** 211-224

Dendrick GS, Sizer PS, Sawyer PG, Brismee JM and Smith MP (2011) Immunohistochemical study of human costotransverse joints. *Clin Anat* **25** 741-747

Erwin WH, Jackson PC and Homonko DA (2000) Innervation of the human costovertebral joint. Implications for clinical back pain syndromes. *J Manipulative Physiol Ther* **23** 395-403

Garcia-Cosamalon J, del Valle ME, Calavia MG, Garcia-Suarez O, Lopez-Muniz A, Otero J and Vega JA (2010) Intervertebral disc, sensory nerves and neurotrophins: who is who in discogenic pain? *J Anat* **217** 1-15

Harris PF and Ranson C (2008) Back and Spine p 29. In *Living and Surface Anatomy for Sports Medicine*. Churchill Livingstone, Edinburgh

Hides J, Stanton W, Mendis MD and Gildea J (2011) Effect of stabilisation training on trunk muscle size, motor control, low back pain and player availability among elite Australian rules football players. *Br J Sports Med* **45** 320

Lederman E (2011) The fall of the postural-structural-biomechanical model in manual and physical therapies: exemplified by lower back pain. *The Journal of Bodywork and Movement Therapies* **15** 131-138

Myers TW (2008) *Anatomy Trains*. 2nd ed.: Churchill Livingstone

Nattiv A, Loucks AB, Manore MM, Sanborn CF, Sundgot-Borgen J and Warren MP (2007) American College of Sports Medicine position stand. The female athlete triad. *Med Sci Sports Exerc* **39** 1867-82

Nitz AJ and Peck D (1986) Comparison of muscle spindle concentrations in large and small human epaxial muscles acting in parallel combinations. *Am Surg* **52** 273-277

Orchard JW, Farhart P and Leopold C (2004) Lumbar spine region pathology and hamstring and calf injuries in athletes: is there a connection. *Br J Sports Med* **38** 502-504

Perich D, Burnett A, O'Sullivan P and Perkin C (2011) Low back pain in adolescent female rowers: a multi-dimensional intervention study. *Knee Surgery, Sports Traumatology, Arthroscopy : Official Journal of the ESSKA* **19**, 20-29

Ranson C, Kerslake R, Burnett A, Batt M and Abdi S (2005) Magnetic resonance imaging of the lumbar spine of asymptomatic professional fast bowlers in cricket. *J Bone Joint Surg Br* **87-B** 1111-1116

Ranson CA, Burnett AF and Kerslake RW (2010) Injuries to the lower back in elite fast bowlers: acute stress changes on MRI predict stress fracture. *The Journal of Bone and Joint Surgery. British Volume* **92**, 1664-1668

Reeves NP, Narendra KS and Cholewicki J (2011) Spine stability: Lessons from balancing a stick. *Clin Biomech* **26** 325-30

Schollum ML, Robertson PA and Broom ND (2009) A microstructural investigation of intervertebral disc lamellar connectivity: detailed analysis of the translamellar bridges. *J Anat* **214** 805-16

Wilke HJ, Neef P, Caimi M, Hoogland T and Claes LE (1999) New in vivo measurements of pressures in the intervertebral disc in daily life. *Spine (Phila Pa 1976)* **24** 755-62

Young BA. Gill HE, Wainner RS and Flynn TW (2008) Thoracic costo-transverse joint pain patterns: A study in normal volunteers. *BMC Musculoskeletal Disord* **9**, 140

Answers

Problem No. 1

i) Thoracic paravertebral muscles
Thoracic joints
Intervertebral
Facet
Costo-vertebral
Costo – transverse
Thoracic Intervertebral disc
Thoracic vertebra
Thoracic nerve roots
Rib
Supraspinous, posterior longitudinal and interspinous ligaments

ii) Cumulative micro-trauma from repetitive high intensity asymmetrical stress on the structures listed above

iii) T6 or T7

iv) May predispose to bony pathology e.g. stress fracture

v) Rib stress fracture

vi) Increased mid-thoracic kyphosis and scoliosis concave to the left due to prolonged right side-flexion in a rower whose oar is on the right.

vii) Associated irritation of the adjacent thoracic sympathetic ganglion

Problem No. 2

i) Pars Interarticularis/Pedicle L3-5
Left L3-S1 facet joints
Paraspinal muscles – Quadratus lumborum and Psoas
Intervertebral disc

ii) Cumulative micro-trauma from repeated end range, high force lumbar extension coupled with left side-flexion and rotation

iii) Pars Interarticularis/Pedicle L3-5 stress fracture
Left L3-S1 facet joint injury
Intervertebral disc

iv) No pain with lumbar flexion
No pain with sitting/coughing/sneezing
Only painful with throwing
No radiating pain
No neurological symptoms

v) Pain only with throwing and extension
Pain eases with a short rest from aggravating activity but resumes soon after

vi) Pain with or without ROM limitation with lumbar extension
Positive Stork test (combined extension, side-flexion and rotation)
Tenderness over the L4 articular pillar
Negative neurological and neural tension tests

vii) Fast bowling in cricket
Pitching in baseball
Golf swing
Tennis serve

viii) MRI – to exclude acute bony stress (marrow oedema, periostitis +/- fracture line in pars interarticularis or pedicle), to exclude joint and disc pathology, to exclude ligamentous or muscular pathology
CT to stage any suspected bony lesion

Problem No. 3

i) L5/S1 Intervertebral disc postero-lateral prolapse

ii) Nerve root

iii) Uncontrolled flexion of the lumbar spine under heavy axial load

iv) Pain with coughing or sneezing due to increased intra-thecal pressure
Weakness of leg and ankle muscles
Pins & Needles or paraesthesia in the leg and foot

v) L 5 / or L4

vi) Tibialis anterior, Peroneus longus and brevis, Hamstrings

vii) Antero-lateral leg and dorsal-medial foot

viii) Hamstring

ix) L4 root compression due to a very lateral L4/5 disc protrusion

Problem No. 4

i) Fracture of any of the left posterior bony elements of the lower cervical spine e.g. transverse process, pedicle, lamina
Compression injury to one or more left lower cervical facet joints
Compression injury to one or more left lower nerve root
ii) Traction injury to the right brachial plexus. Often known as a 'stinger' injury
iii) C5 - Deltoid - Resisted shoulder abduction
C6 - Biceps – Resisted elbow flexion

T1 - Adductor pollicis – Resisted thumb adduction
iv) C7 - Skin over palmar and dorsal 3rd finger
   C6 - Lateral forearm
   C8 - Medial hand and postero-medial forearm
v) C6/7 facet joint compression injury
vi) Deep neck flexor muscles
   Anterior longitudinal ligament
   Strain injury due to the forceful cervical extension

Problem No. 5

i) Commonly see increase in pre-dental space on lateral X-radiograph if transverse ligament is damaged and displacement of C1 lateral masses on odontoid.
ii) Computed Tomography to obtain a 3D appreciation of the bony architecture
iii) The loss of C1-2 bony congruency and potential disruption of the transverse ligament may leave the injured person with the sensation that their head might 'fall off'.
iv) Tackling in American Football when the tackler dives forwards and plants the top of his helmet against the body of an opponent
v) C1/2 facet joints
   Sub-occipital muscles

Problem No. 6

i) That play is stopped so the player and first aider staff are safe
   That the player has a patent airway and his breathing and circulation are stable
ii) Manual in-line stabilisation (MILS) of the cervical spine
iii) Using a spinal board and collar
iv) Posterior cervical ligament complex
   Dorsal cervical paraspinal muscles
   Cervical vertebrae
   Disc
   Spinal cord
v) C5
vi) Computed Tomography

Problem No. 7

i) Anterior wedge compression vertebral fracture
ii) A higher risk of decreased bone density in females of this age
iii) Thoracic facet joints
   Costo-vertebral and costo-transverse joints
   Posterior longitudinal ligament
   Erector spinae musculature
   Thoracic intervertebral disc

Problem No. 8

i) As an Indy Car racer the driver's neck musculature would be conditioned to controlling only left hand turns and may not be sufficiently developed to safely control the neck against the G forces associated with sharp right hand turns on touring car circuits.

ii) Rotation 90°
Side Flexion

iii) Painful inhibition of cervical muscles
Dysfunction of one or more cervical facet joints (due to sprain or spondylosis)
Cervical muscle spasm involving Upper trapezius, Splenius capitis, rectus capitus major and minor, semispinalis capitis, levator scapulae, sternocledomastoidius, superior and inferior oblique

iv) Chronic neck injury due to previous car racing accidents
Cumulative joint, disc and soft tissue micro-trauma due to the G forces associated with high speed cornering

v) C6 nerve root dysfunction

vi) Cervical disc protrusion compressing the nerve root within the spinal canal
Foraminal stenosis due to osteophytes, or ligamentous hypertrophy particularly the ligamentum flavum.

vii) Median nerve

Problem No. 9

i) Erector spinae

ii) Left quadratus lumborum
Lateral erector spine e.g. ilio-costalis or longissimus thoracis

iii) T10/11 facet (zygapophyseal) joint
Eleventh rib costo-transverse and costo-vertebral joints

iv) Eleventh rib fracture or stress fracture
Costo-transverse or costo-vertebral joint sprain

v) Rib compression

vi) To exclude haematuria that might indicate kidney damage

Index